BEYOND

BEYOND WORDS

Interpretive Art Therapy

JOHANNES S. BODTKER

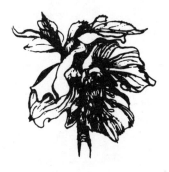

Clunie Press
for
The Roland Harris Trust Library
Monograph Series No. 4

© The Roland Harris Education Trust 1990
ISBN 902 965 27 1
First Published 1990

All rights reserved. No part of this publication may be reproduced, stored in a retrieval system, or transmitted, in any form or by any means, electronic, mechanical, photocopying, recording, or otherwise, without the prior permission of The Roland Harris Education Trust.

Printed and bound in Great Britain by
Billing & Sons Ltd, Worcester

Contents

	Introduction	1
1	Bluebird	23
2	Rocket	53
3	Black Rhomb	73
4	Eagle	89
5	Punishing Iron	109
	Illustrations	129

Introduction

Art interpreting therapy is a form of psychoanalytically oriented psychotherapy. The basic element is art produced through painting or drawing in the therapy sessions.[1] The method was developed through therapeutic work with children and adolescents presenting with neurotic, psychotic and developmental disturbances.

The method is based on Freud's main work, "Traumdeutung" (The Interpretation of Dreams); his method of free association and psychoanalysis; modified child-analysis and psychoanalytically oriented play therapy.

There are several special problems connected with child psychotherapy: a) children prefer action to verbalization; b) they prefer externalizing to introspection when it comes to solving problems; c) the method of free association is not easily adapted to child analysis; d) many children have a low tolerance to the painful and anxiety-provoking effects of psychotherapy. Also, children do not often make their own decisions about beginning, continuing, or completing treatment. All of these factors are interrelated.

By introducing play into the therapy situation, child therapists were able to overcome some of the difficulties mentioned above. Nevertheless, I have often found play therapy to be unsatisfactory because it lacks a medium that will ensure a continuous creative process.[2]

Although child analysis has some unfavourable aspects, it is not without advantages. A child's personality is developing all the time, problems have been allowed to influence the child's psychological structure for a limited time only, and the possible effects of problems on character development are thus less pronounced. The tendency to intellectualize is not as developed in children, leaving their feelings more accessible than in most adults. Their dreams in particular are less distorted by efforts to condense and displace issues, and consequently their latent dream wishes are easier to interpret.[3] A state of transference is often established fairly easily with children; it is not usually marred by scepticism and will often be quite profound.

Several psychotherapists and art therapists have based their work on art, and two different branches of art therapy have emerged:

One, in which painting and drawing are valued for their creative aspect. The picture in itself becomes the central object, and the therapeutic effect lies in the creative process. Psychotherapeutic interpretation is not a factor here.

Another, which is based on the child's own interpretations of the pictures. These interpretations, in addition to the emotional involvement in the pictorial content within a transference situation and the creative aspect of the activity, constitute the central issues in this form of therapy, and not the product itself.

Both these branches of therapy are called "Art therapy", — the former is also referred to as "Picture therapy" or "Paint-therapy".

A classic therapist within the former branch of art therapy is Edith Kramer. She outlines her therapeutic work thus:

> "The starting point is the creative artist and the educationist with a Freudian way of thinking. The emphasis, however, is on the idea of art as therapy rather than a psychotherapy where art is used as a tool ... art therapy is most of all to be perceived as an aid to support the client's ego, nurse a feeling of identity and encourage the maturation process in general. Its main function lies in the ability of art to contribute to the development of a psychological organization which can function under external pressure without breaking down, without the patient finding it necessary to escape into inhibiting defence mechanisms."

This form of therapy is used independently or as a supplement to psychotherapy.

Margaret Naumburg is one of the classics within the other form of art therapy. She describes her starting point thus:

> "Spontaneous drawings as products of the imagination are satisfactions of wishes — this manifest content (the drawings), probably always in some respects covers or disguises unconscious underlying motives — expresses problems involving certain 'polarities', e.g. life-death, male-

female, father-mother, love-hate, activity-passivity ... graphic art affords the opportunity to project all of these trends extensively."

About the method she says:

"The process of liberation into 'free' expression in art cannot take place by merely urging the patient to make whatever he wishes, he must first gain confidence and discover his ability to do so. Artistic technique is not ignored but is introduced in an incidental manner after the patient has begun to express himself. — By 'free' art expression is meant an authentic and original response to life (either inner or outer), made in some chosen art form ... The term 'free' art expression (is) not absolute or unconditioned. Every individual is conditioned by factors working upon him from both within and without ... among dominant influences ... from the environment are those related to general cultural and economic milieu, the parental attitudes, the school experiences ..."

About the implementation, she says:

"When the patient has been helped to overcome his inhibitions and is able to express his deepest fears, wishes and fantasies on paper ... he is tapping the unconscious in the symbolic language of images, which will often bring to the surface what he dares not or cannot say in words ..."

Her method is based on letting the patients interpret their own pictures —

"no interpretations are given — for to the writer the therapeutic value of such expressions does not depend on interpretation, but rather on its value as an image language of the unconscious ..."

In her practical work, however, she takes an active part in the interpretation, for instance in the treatment of a schizophrenic girl, 18 years old:

"Thus the patients own responses to her symbolic dream pictures were *reformulated** so as to point out to her the revealing significance of her own comments ..." (**My underlining*. JSB)

BEYOND WORDS

ART INTERPRETING THERAPY

In the light of the particular problems and advantages involved in child therapy, it seems natural to include a child's dreams and day dreams as expressed through painting and drawing in the therapeutic work. The language of art becomes an important tool in the interpretation of a child's dream content. Thus one escapes to a certain extent (see p. 20 "Psychotherapeutic Interpretation") the problems connected with free verbal association in child therapy and the child's preference for action becomes a creative rather than obstructive factor, allowing for the expression of multidetermined dream elements.[4]

By asking for pictorial responses to the various elements of a manifest, dream-related picture, one obtains a pictorial expression of the condensing and displacing efforts that such dream-related pictures are a result of. Eventually one obtains simple, graphic pictorial expressions of the latent dream wishes or derivatives of these.

I begin in art-interpreting therapy by urging the patient to "free" art expression. As Margaret Naumburg pointed out, a "free" art production is limited by what the child has already learnt about drawing and painting — and it may be quite a while before it is able to produce a picture which is entirely its own. My challenge to free art expression often needs to be repeated — my usual comment being, "Paint whatever comes to your mind — the important thing is that it's YOUR picture, not something you've seen elsewhere. It doesn't have to be great art!"

In addition to free picture production, I have at times found it desirable to encourage the child to a graphic clarification of a particular theme or motif. This is true especially where the child's relationship to its internalized mother[5] or to the transference situation is concerned. In such a case, I often show the child an earlier picture which is especially representative of the actual situation, and I ask the child to clarify the theme by painting another picture. This is what I call a "prompted" picture.

Another version of "prompted" pictures is the kind of pictures I get when I ask for graphic associations to a single motif in a given picture. Often a child has created a multi-determined composition containing a representation of her relationship to her father, her mother, and jealousy of her siblings. Such a picture is produced as a link in a chain of pictures. I will select the part of such a picture which I feel represents or covers a detail which is of special therapeutic interest. The underlying problem must be preconscious or on the verge of becoming conscious. Experience shows that this form of guidance does not disturb a natural development of the therapeutic process, but rather enhances it.

The method of combining the use of free art expression and prompted pictures is anchored in the theory of the psychoanalytical interpretation of dreams, which thus becomes the model for this method. The pictures which I elect to treat in this manner must have a day dream or dream-related quality, and may thus be compared to the manifest dream. When I ask for a pictorial association to a particular motif in a picture, this may similarly be compared to the psychoanalytical challenge to associate verbally to parts of a dream. Often I will receive a combination of pictorial and verbal associations.

Chapter 1, Bluebird, contains such a sequence, in the part where the big lion enters the scene, (see p. 16, Narrative). As in a dream, we may deduce that the main character is the person who painted the picture. The lion is Bluebird herself, and Bluebird is aware of this. (This is her 30th therapy session. She knows that the pictures represent something in her own mind.) The endeavour to distort reality is apparent in that the oral attack shifts from the sister to the former teacher, then to a classmate. The unfolding of the real situation occurred when I asked for associations to "the little bunny", then to "the long-short mane". A masculine symbol, a horse, is used here to camouflage the fact that the person in question is her sister. The lilac bow on the horse's tail is a clear indication that this is so — basically I regard the bow as "a slip of the tongue", confirming that the horse represents a female person. That the attack is oral, also indicates that it is aimed at the mother. Thus the big, open mouth represents a doubly determined attack — against the sister who took the mother from her, and against the mother who let this happen. (The above concerns itself solely with sibling rivalry and should be regarded as only a part of the interpretation.) Thus prompted pictures represent a guided part of an otherwise spontaneous production of unique pictures.

In addition to the challenge to free art expression and prompted pictures, I use three other forms of intervention:

a) a graphic clarification, that is, analysis of how the graphic elements are employed in the picture;
b) an expressionistic clarification, that is, analysis of what is being expressed by the picture;
c) a psychotherapeutic interpretation, that is, a comment on the fulfilment of wishes which the picture reflects.

The three kinds of intervention listed above may be utilized in this order when, for instance, I analyze a dream-related picture sequence. However, my graphic clarification may become superfluous as soon as the child masters the use of graphic elements. Even the expressionistic clarification may be taken over by the child when it has learned, in the course of therapy, to express itself fluently in the language of art.

Heavy resistance from the child's censoring agent may interfere with such development. When this happens, I may have to start over with thorough graphic clarification, often through several sessions, before the child allows me, or can manage itself, to attach any expressive content to the strokes, forms or colors presented in a picture.

GRAPHIC CLARIFICATION

The graphic elements are my first concern in the analysis. The formal graphic elements are: line, color and color value. A *line* can be short or long, straight or curved, with a sharp or a soft angle. Furthermore, a line can be horizontal or vertical, diagonal or radial; all quantities that can be measured.

The second element is *color value*, that is, all degrees between black and white, brilliance of light and shadow. This indicates the weight of the picture or accent of the motif. We may see delicate pencil lines, like in the drawings of "Iron", Chapter 6, picture nos. 25/26, his last session, where for the first time he draws a human figure according to his own experience of being a human. This picture is almost weightless — it could be erased with a single stroke. Compare this with picture no. 15 in the

INTRODUCTION

same chapter — the picture of his evil companion, where he has painted the head-symbol coal-black. To him, the latter picture has annihilating weight.

The third element, *color*, gives the picture its quality. "It lends to salt its saltiness and to sugar its sweetness." (Paul Klee, 1924). Color, in other words, gives identity to otherwise similar objects. (Further enlargement on color follows below under the description of expressionistic clarification).

Secondly, my graphic comments are based on how the three formal elements are employed in *form*: scribble, compositions, or sketches; in *direction*: right, left, centrifugal, centripetal, or diagonal; in *movement*: broken up, continuous, circular or undulating; and *rhythm*: intervals, length, accent, etc.

The composition of a picture may be *simple*, as in the last picture of a sequence during the analysis of a dream-related picture. It may stand for a death wish or a derivative of such (id-derivative). See for instance Chapter 1, Bluebird, in the picture of the planet car driver and the deadly bomb (picture no. 30), where the bomb threatening the car driver represents the death wish, in the transference situation aimed at the therapist, the car driver. The composition is produced in a dreamy state of mind, is sketchy, monovalent and monochromatic.

Bluebird's picture no. 7, *The Viking Spoil*, is a carefully composed theme. In its entirety, the composition presents the oedipal situation, camouflaged as a viking raid. It is divided into a father-theme with the church and the phallus-steeple and a mother-theme with the vaulted hut containing treasure. The main theme, the raid, is *presented* in the center of the picture, in a vehement rhythm, by the vikings' rush to the shore; *carried out* through the vikings' stealing the treasure from the lower part of the mother-building, the vaulted hut, in a subdued, seductive rhythm, and *concluding* with the burning of the ships at the far right, in a dissolving rhythm.

A more conscious effort is Eagle's picture no. 6 of her bulimia-situation. The theme is reproduced in a strict, premeditated composition; it is clearly bipartite, consisting of a vertical, fencing element to the left, and a circular maelstrom to the right. Here is a double rhythm: the regular vertical lines to the left with an excluding, prohibiting effect, and to the right, a grinding, circular movement towards the center, like an engulfing mael-strom, a picture of the *circulus vitiosus* that is bulimia.

The therapeutic intention of the graphic clarification is to make the child aware that it is *she* who creates something through the use of graphic elements — that no line is accidental, that this kind of communication is a language — the language of art.

The expressionistic content in a child's work of art is a result of how the technical aspect is approached, particularly at the start of therapy. Initially, a child will often deny that the graphic part of a picture has an expressionistic correlate. The first time you ask a 6 year old child who has painted a red and blue flower what it is supposed to be, he may answer, "it is a red and blue flower," period! After you have offered a graphic description of how he has used the pictorial options, the expressive content may gradually gain the quality of having been experienced, and he may say spontaneously, "It's a warm, sunny day and I'm looking forward to going away to the country." Thus a clarification of the graphic content may have the effect of making conscious the expressionistic content of a picture.

EXPRESSIONISTIC CLARIFICATION

An expressionistic clarification is analysis and accentuation of the pictorial expression. The expressive content of a picture consists of the thoughts, feelings, or notions' which it is intended to convey.

The picture may consist of a simple motif or it may be composed of several motifs to form a theme.

The theme may be more or less complex, and one single picture may present several themes originating from different levels of consciousness.

The pictorial expression may be explicit or implicit, disguised or exposed, declaratory or merely hinted at; it may be embellished with idyllic, diversionary decorations, or brutally amplified by startling color values and a cut-up rhythm, like cracks in ice or broken glass.

I base the expressionistic clarification on how the graphic elements are utilized to lend expression to the picture and my comment will therefore often be of a complex nature. One example of this is Bluebird's picture no. 53. I have asked her to draw mother, and receive one of her characteristic, sketchy, spontaneous pictures. The expression in this picture is a product of the interaction between my graphic/expressionistic comments and her explanations. Because I say, 'elongated arm', for instance, she says 'pulls my hair', the graphic/expressionistic factor conveys and amplifies the experienced content. By accentuating the term 'elongated' (which belongs in the graphic category), I implicitly convey that the arm is expressing something forceful (which belongs in the expressionistic category). Her answer, 'pulls my hair', has the quality of being experienced. Thus the whole picture gains the quality of having been experienced, which is the purpose of pictorial clarification.

Sometimes it is difficult to establish a flow of pictorial/experience-related communication. This is true of Black Rhomb's picture no. 2. I have asked her to think 'mother' for this picture (see Black Rhomb, Narrative, p. 3). Here I have to describe the black rhomb and particularly the central bright yellow patch to show that the picture not only represents mother, but also, and especially, the longing for mother.[7] So also with the three tiny, red "fuzzy balls". They had to be described as "tiny" before she could accept that they also longed for contact with mother.

Color Analysis
Colors, their combination and nuances, lend the picture its quality. Color analysis is therefore a particularly important part of the expressionistic clarification. A particular color often represents the same feeling or motif to many different children. Still, the patient's individual color scheme should always be established as soon as possible in a therapy, because people who are central in the patient's environment are often represented by a distinct color in the patient's mind. Below is a list of what the various colors *often* stand for.

Red: often stands for hatred or love, intense feelings, blood, sexual anxiety, and is often combined with black to enhance the anxiety provoking aspect.
Yellow: often stands for longing, searching, warmth or light.

Green:	stands for fertility, growth.
Orange:	often stands for fertility. Combined with red: fire, consuming love. Combined with brown: something perishable or transitory.
Blue:	often stands for clarity, purity, loftiness, sensibility, transcendency.
Violet:	often represents something sad, resigned. Combined with different pastels: personal integration, sublimated conflict.
Brown:	often represents mess or dirt, excrement. Combined with green and yellow, germination or fertilization.

Mixed colors, like turquoise, may stand for personal integration, often combined with pink and various pastels. A structured *design* of colors, like a rainbow, may stand for family conflict or a bridge between contrasting feelings. I have left out black and white, since these are not colors. Black and white are most often used to add weight to an issue, to indicate values. *Black* may represent annihilation, oppression, anxiety, isolation; *white* may represent undefined, unknown, weightless qualities or it may represent the failure of something to be present (unknown parent, a resolved oedipal conflict, frigidity, impotence, emptiness, etc.).

CLASSIFICATION OF PICTURES

Gradually, through practising art interpreting therapy, I have found that the various pictures may be organized into three different categories. The criteria for classification are: (a) graphic composition: construction, complex design or simple detail; (b) expressive content: complex, carefully composed theme or single motif; (c) state of mind at the time of execution: contemplative, daydreamy, or dreamy.

Pictures which are characterized by the first alternatives under (a), (b), and (c) belong in the first category; pictures which fit into the second group of alternatives belong in the second category, and so on.

Below is a description of the pictures in the three categories:

1. In the first category, one gets the clearly conscious, pre-

meditated constructions. Often they are somewhat elaborate, marked by a far-fetched combination of single motifs, and embellished with, for instance, idyllic field flowers or marred by grossly exaggerated, uncalled for, details. Both variations are there to divert attention from and camouflage the central motif. It is essential to analyse such pictures graphically and expressionistically with the child to be able to uncover and understand the central theme and the various individual motifs.

In short, in this category one will find elaborate constructions with a complex expressive content, created in a contemplative state of mind.

2. In the second category, in the middle range of pictures, I find spontaneous, skilful compositions that are produced compulsively, prompted by an inner, irresistible urge (see Freud's term: "compulsion to repeat") in a daydream-related emotional state. These pictures have several interrelated motifs combined to form a single theme. They are produced quickly with confident brush strokes. The single motifs are well defined, as is the theme's outline. The time and place of action are often rearranged: for instance the time may be "before there were people in the world", and the place may be far away, like "in Africa". The main character is often camouflaged, for instance as another person: "viking-chief", "truck-driver", or as a symbol: "an arrow," "a volcano," etc., but is always the picture's originator.

The rhythm is often complex, dual or triple. One motif may be painted in a light, dancing, seductive rhythm, another in a vehement, intrusive, and persistent rhythm. Between the two one finds incantations of an embellishing, camouflaging and consequently diversionary kind. Often the colors merge to an organic unity, lending a multivocal, yet clarified quality to the motifs and the theme. One seldom finds gross discords here, and the total picture may leave an impression similar to that of a musical fugue. Such pictures reflect the "artist's" pre-conscious.

In short, in the above category one will find compound compositions with a well defined expressive theme, created in a daydreamy state of mind under the sway of an infantile urge.

3. In the third kind of picture, at the far end of the range, the child projects unconscious, dream-related, quickly sketched, transitory single motifs. Seemingly prompted by infantile impulses, these pictures will emerge like sunbeams through an opening in the clouds. They are monocrome, and monovalent.

The dominant feature may be a *person* disguised as "a witch", "a chinese woman," etc., or an *act*, symbolized by the throwing of a bomb, a stealing hand, etc. They are handed to the therapist in the same resolute manner in which they are produced, whereupon the child starts on another motif, or a diversionary 'butterfly-picture' of a more technical-experimental character.

In short, in the above category one will find simple sketches with distinct single motifs, produced in a dreamy state of mind and prompted by infantile impulses.

A *sequence* of pictures from a therapeutic session may consist of pictures from the three categories as follows. The sequence may begin with a conscious construction, Category 1., leaping to a well-composed fugal theme, Category 2., through picture-association to a motif, whereupon it may arrive at an unconscious, sketchy single motif, Category 3., through further association to a small detail like for instance "the long-short mane" of Bluebird's "stupid horse" (picture no. 18). A sketch of this kind at the end of a picture sequence may reflect an impulse under primary repression or a derivative of such an impulse.

PSYCHOTHERAPEUTIC INTERPRETATION

As regards interpretation of the infantile material that emerges in an art-interpreting therapy, I follow the rules laid down in the theory of child analysis. I shall describe some of the features that particularly pertain to the art interpreting form of therapy.

The initial child-physician relationship, typical of any therapy, is often of short duration. At this stage it is essential to elicit the child's curiosity, especially with regard to graphic potential.

INTRODUCTION

When the child experiences that her art work reflects important issues in her mind, the ground is laid for an exploration/guidance situation.

Bluebird experienced her role as an explorer fully in her 27th session (picture no. 12), where she presented herself as a rocket about to explore the world, and myself as a magnifying glass which is going to show her the way and warn her about danger. Even though she did not surrender to being in the position of explorer rather than patient until the 27th session, we see from her third picture, *The Mysterious Lake*, that preconsciously she sensed at an early stage that the pictures concerned herself.

Whether or not the basis for interpretation exists is dependent on whether or not a transference relationship has been established. In art interpreting therapy the transference situation is usually established fairly easily and will soon develop into a deep relationship. In my opinion, this is due to the inherent creative potential of the medium and the tools — the pencils, crayons, paint in many different colors, and brushes. The artistic material makes it possible for the dream image to be projected without translation into verbal language.
[8] The expressive potential implicit in the artistic material seems to be experienced by the child at an early stage of the treatment.

This does not mean that verbalization is to be ignored, but that it is important that the child is initially offered a medium to project her dream image as it is conceived, without having to translate it. The dream material that is to be projected may be of a very complex nature. Described in artistic terms, a daydream-related picture, when projected, may look like and be interpreted as a multivocal fugal composition with several single motifs, with different rhythms. The expressive content may reflect, as in Bluebird's picture no. 2, a threefold situation: her actual class situation, the relationship to her sister, and her oedipal conflict. To demand a primary verbalization of this material in its entirety is not realistic, and it would be very difficult, if not impossible, to reproduce it in any form other than an artistic or mythical one.

In brief, art as a creative medium enhances the transference relationship, and an artistic projection of the complex material of a therapy ensures a wide range of re-living. ("Wide range of re-living" is here used both in the sense of including related issues from different areas of life, and re-living of the issues on different levels of consciousness.)

NEGATIVE TRANSFERENCE

Negative transference usually represents a difficult though crucial stage in any therapeutic process. In art interpreting therapy negative transference takes place in an artistic, muted and externalized form. Nevertheless, the content of the transference is both a re-living of a part of the child's inner reality, and a current experience in relation to the therapist.[9] In my view, the specific therapeutic effect is based on the wide range of re-lived experiences made possible by a creative medium. One aspect only of a multidetermined theme may be verbalized, either by the child itself or by me, as an interpretation, but the related aspects implicit in the created picture are also influenced by the interpretation. It is justifiable, I believe, to regard this therapeutic influence as a cluster-effect.[10]

The use of a creative medium also seems to act as an insurance against the most difficult resistance phenomena, like excessive outbursts or attempts to terminate the treatment.

One example of negative transference is expressed in Bluebird's Planet car driver sequence, pictures 26–29. Her death-wish is here transferred to the therapist by projecting a deadly bomb onto the picture, placed right underneath the therapist, the planet car driver. The fact that she verbally had to reduce the effect into "injured, not dead, with a very poor life," seems only to prove that the wish was experienced as deadly.

Another example is to be found in the narrative of Punishing Iron in the part where he is throwing up the iron. This symbolic action is presented in pictures no. 20 and 21. Punishing Iron is externalizing his cruel, annihilating superego through drawing and miming. The symbol of the punishing element, the iron, is transferred to me by throwing it up into my open hands, for safer storage. Because of his previous painting of the punishing superego-symbol, he has made it possible for me to comply with his wish to transfer the annihilating iron to me. The act of throwing out his cruel super-ego (the iron) is probably followed by a re-introjection of a modified super-ego. The annihilating

INTRODUCTION

quality of the iron is transformed by the therapist's receiving it unharmed, thus demonstrating its non-deadly character.

ARCHAIC UTERINE SYMBOLS

The archaic uterus-symbols which are presented in several pictures that are created in art interpreting therapy are of special therapeutic interest.

> One example is Iron's picture no. 20. The uterine symbol here is a round shape made up of circular strokes with blank areas between the strokes. It is a dirty yellow color and its tone value is light. The immediate impression is that this is a somewhat sketchy cave. From this "cave", Iron "chases Daddy out of Mommy", while appropriating the contents of the uterine cavity.
>
> Another example is Eagle's pictures no. 10–12. In picture no. 10 the archaic symbol is formed like a narrow indentation, filled in with multicolored dots, in a vertical, black composition. In the 11th picture the motif is further elaborated to form a similar indentation, lined with green, assaulted by a brown brush stroke, with heavy black horizontal strokes to underline the destruction of the uterine content.
>
> In picture no. 12 she develops the motif even further. The result is a double composition: First, a peripheral circle symbolizes the uterine cavity, or, as she puts it, "the embracing mother." The mother figure is lying down at the lower part of the circle, with the upper part symbolizing "the embrace." Second, a central black form with dense arrows points at the mother figure, symbolizing the assault on her mother's body.
>
> A third example is Black Rhomb's picture no. 33. The composition is outlined in black and consists of an upper part, a head, and a lower part, the body. Inside the body is placed "a dragon that spits fire," in the shape of a red lump, underneath which are red and yellow flames radiating from a black core. This scene symbolizes herself inside her mother's womb attempting to liberate herself.
>
> These three examples all deal with attempted assaults on the

uterus. In the first example, Iron is chasing daddy out of mommy. This happens in an annihilating dimension and the effect on the development is catastrophic. In the second example, Eagle's narrow indentation and embracing mother, the assault takes place in a dimension of ambivalence and has a splitting effect on her mind. In the third example, Black Rhomb's firespitting dragon, the scene takes place in a liberating dimension, and has a supportive effect on her struggle towards individuation.

Assaults on uterine contents as revealed in these archaic pictures are described by Melanie Klein in her studies on the earliest stages of the oedipal development.[11] To her, the excessive hatred which develops in early infancy is due to the occurence of the first oedipal conflict at a time when the infant cannot speak or understand what is being said and is simultaneously dominated by the anal-sadistic stage of psycho-sexual development. These circumstances lead to a wish to appropriate the contents of the mother's body.

The archaic motifs projected in the above mentioned pictures, are precisely of the kind which Melanie Klein describes, originating in the early oedipal conflict and occurring during the anal-sadistic stage of psycho-sexual development. Art interpreting therapy offers a child the possibility of re-living, in a transference relationship, its earliest experiences of privation,[12] using a creative, pictorial mode. The process of re-living probably has a therapeutic effect even without any explicit interpretation at this archaic level. Often an interpretation of the derivative meaning on a pre-conscious level will reveal the archaic meaning (cluster-effect.) This effect does not reveal itself in relation to the single interpretation, but in the long-term development of the therapy. I regard this as an example of Lacan's (1936) concept of "the two forms of time:" the "moments of truth" (the interpretations,) and the "time of understanding" (the treatment process). The child and the therapist are both engaged in this twofold process of time. On the other hand, an interpretation at this archaic level may be meaningful for the child, and may be "encircled by words"[13] by the therapist, if both are in true contact with this narcissistic, pre-verbal area of painful functioning. This process is described in the narrative of Iron, picture no. 20, and in the narrative of Black Rhomb, picture no. 33.

Thus, in my opinion, this mode of re-living in the transference situation — with or without interpretation — constitutes the main reason why art interpreting therapy can establish contact with, and ease the pain of, the often therapy-resistant conditions following early privation.

Notes to Introduction

1. Psychoanalysis, and most forms of dynamic psychotherapy (or "psychoanalytically oriented psychotherapy") are commonly thought of as a "talking cure" (as formulated by Breuer's patient Anna O.) More recently, Lacan[1] has stated (see list of references: Svein Haugsgjerd: "Jacques Lacan og psychoanalysen," p. 45, 1986) that psychoanalysis is a "process which takes place in the spoken language, and nowhere else". He describes the analysand's stream of words as a chain of "signifiers", vehicles of meaning. In art interpreting therapy the sequences of paintings covering specific themes function as such chains of signifiers, as far as their expressionistic content is transformed into words, either by the child or the therapist.
2. James S. Grotstein ("Who is the Dreamer Who Dreams the Dream and who is the Dreamer Who Understands It?) 1979, from "Do I Dare Disturb the Universe?" 1981:
   "*Phantasy* functions through splitting the chaotic data into recognizable qualities of separateness (pleasurable and unpleasurable, etc.). The elements are then separated into "objects" of convenience. The establishment of the separated objects constitutes an act of *creation* of essential phantasies."
3. Anna Freud, in "Normality and Pathology in Childhood", (1966) pp. 14-15, points to the
   "simple fulfilment dreams (of children) which reveal the underlying wishes; there are also the conscious day dreams which give information about the day dreamer's libidinal development with minimal distortions."
   She emphasizes that this material is a derivative of the unconscious and must not be mistaken for "unconscious material proper".

4. "Bion's conception of alpha-function is a mythical mechanism which accounts for our activity to concentrate attention by day and by night (to be able to concentrate on being attentively awake and focusing by day, and "attentive to sleep by night.") The dream therefore helps us to handle stimuli which is quantitatively and qualitatively excessive so that a membrane of alpha-elements can separate sleep from wakefulness, unconsciousness from consciousness, etc." (Quoted from James S. Grotstein: Who is the Dreamer?, 1979).
I interpret the mythic material projected in dream related paintings according to Grotstein's conceptions to which I am only able to refer briefly here.
5. "Internalized" objects is a concept which is described in object relation theory (Klein.) An internalized object is thought to be the infant's unconscious, pre-verbal inner image of mother/father as it evolves in the early oedipal stage during the first year of life. Such images are the result not only of the parents' conscious/unconscious feelings and attitudes, but also of a wide range of social, cultural, and economic conditions or of physical afflictions.
6. Wilfrid Bion, "A Theory of Thinking" (Article in *Learning from Experience* (1962):
"The infant is born with pre-conceptions or "empty thoughts", for instance the vague notion of a feeding breast, the mother's womb with a certain content, that there exists a mother-father pair with an intimate relationship from which the infant is excluded ..." (Referred from S. Haugsgjerd, 1986).
(see "The archaic uterine symbols," Introduction, pp. 24)
7. Svein Haugsgjerd: "Grunnlaget for en ny psykiatri," Pax forlag, 1986, p. 334, referring to Jacques Lacan's lecture (1953) on "The field and function of speech and the word":
" — But sometimes, in privileged moments, the conventional connection of speech is broken by a slip of the tongue, a lapse of memory, a funny formulation, a symptom, to put it shortly, something unexpected. Then the unconscious breaks into the speech, and at this moment a revelation may happen — an interpretation. The interpretation may come from the therapist, but just as well

from the analysand, and it is *her or his* word and nothing else which constitutes the origin of the interpretation. In this moment, when the unconscious wish can reveal itself in its truth, the word leaps from an empty sound to a filled word, filled with meaning."

8. Sigmund Freud: Drommetydning II, (*The Interpretation of Dreams*) (1985), p. 65:
"With these considerations (Freud is referring to a dream where the central recollected image was the conductor of an orchestra, standing on a platform on the top of a tall tower in parterre, surrounded by an iron fence . . .) we have at last uncovered a third element with a not insignificant part in the transformation of dream thoughts into dream content: *The concern for the possibility of presenting the peculiar psychic material which the dream utilizes*, for the most part in visual images. Among the various by-products of the main dream thoughts, undoubtedly are preferred those which make possible a visual presentation, and to the dream work, no effort is too great when it comes to remolding a fragile thought into a different mode of expression, even if it means a more unusual one — if only it makes possible the presentation and thus terminates the psychologically strained situation in which the thought process finds itself. Such remolding of thought content into another form may incidentally prove useful also to the work of condensation and establish a relation to a new thought, relations which otherwise would not have been established . . . (Freud's underlining).

9. Donald Meltzer: *Dream Life* (1983) as referred to by Svein Haugsgjerd in "Grunnlaget for en ny psykiatri," p. 360:
"Meltzer illustrates the Kleinian view on transference in this connection: We are not talking about transference from the past to the present, but from inner reality to the interactional relationship between the analysand and analyst."
And:
"Meltzer emphasizes that the analyst must work at, and make a genuine effort the whole time, not only to listen, but also to participate in a dialogue. Kleinians are often reproached for their tendency to set forth too many hasty

and penetrating interpretations, thus influencing or indoctrinating the patient. Meltzer makes it clear, however, that any one interpretation does not have to be the final answer, not even a preliminary one, but an exploratory act: the therapist involves himself in the patient's use of images, offering his own associations — among other things using symbols from the language of child sexuality — thus stimulating the patient to go on in the visualization of his (her) images." (Haugsgjerd on referring to D. Meltzer (1967, p. 357.)

10. In Bion's terms interpretation (either by the child or by the therapist) is an alpha-function. Grotstein ("Who is the Dreamer?, p. 385) writes about the alpha-function:
" — Alpha-function seems able to link up the experience with the archetypes corresponding to it to produce finally a mythic dream narrative sequence which conveys personal meaningfulness to the dreamer (by day and by night.)"
I think my suggested "cluster-effect" could be explained using this description by Grotstein as a model.
Bion elaborates further on this theme: (From *Attention and Interpretation*, 1970):
"Where does the therapy lead us? To change, to growth, to an extended awareness, passions and myths. But only a small part of such an extension may be arrested by words. The psychoanalysis leads to an *absolute* increase in the knowledge of oneself, but also a *relative* decrease, maintains Bion. (My underlining, JSB.) This means that the increase of emotional awareness is much greater than the intellectual one." (Haugsgjerd, 1986, p. 354.)

11. Melanie Klein (1928) "Early stages of the Oedipus conflict" (from '*Contributions to Psychoanalysis*' 1921 – 1945," p. 204:
"We find that important consequences ensue from the fact that the ego is still so little developed when it is assailed by the onset of the Oedipus tendencies and the incipient sexual curiosity associated with them. The infant, still undeveloped intellectually, is exposed to an onrush of problems and questions. One of the most bitter grievances which we come upon in the unconscious is that these many overwhelming questions, which are apparently only partly

conscious, and even when conscious cannot yet be expressed in words, remain unanswered. Another reproach follows hard upon this, namely, that the child could not understand words and speech. Thus the first questions go back beyond the beginnings of his understanding of speech.

In analysis both these grievances give rise to an extraordinary amount of hate. Singly or in conjunction they are the cause of numerous inhibitions of the epistemophilic impulse. The early feeling of *not knowing* has manifold connections. It unites with the feeling of being incapable, impotent, which soon results from the Oedipus situation ... The early connection between the epistemophilic impulse and the sadism is very important for the whole mental development. This instinct, activated by the rise of the Oedipus tendencies, at first mainly concerns itself with *the mother's body*, which is assumed to be the scene of all sexual processes and development. The child is still dominated by the anal-sadistic libido-position which impels him to wish to *appropriate* the contents of her body." (Melanie Klein's underlining.)

12. I prefer to use the term "privation" here instead of conflict, because it seems to be a more adequate term to describe the painful feeling actually experienced in the therapy sessions.
13. Arne Skouen: "What cannot be arrested by words can only be encircled."

1   Bluebird

NARRATIVE

Bluebird was 9 years old when her parents contacted us[1]. The reason for their doing so was Bluebird's increasing problems in school during the previous half year, both in keeping up with her class intellectually and in adjusting socially. She was in the second half of the third grade.

Her mother thought the main reason for her problems might by dyslexia.[2] She was herself educationally oriented. Bluebird's father emphasized her habit of withdrawing into intense games of make-believe. He assumed that her excessive fantasizing was the real reason for her learning disability.

Her teacher felt that she "really was too immature for this class level." She had been advised to wait another year before starting school because she was "under-age and immature", at 6 years and 8 months. Now, in the third grade, she was one year behind intellectually and showed a "strange lack of adjustment in class.".

My advice to her parents was that we arrange for Bluebird to undergo some tests, especially with regard to dyslexia. I also considered it necessary to talk to her teacher and in addition have Bluebird tested by a special ed. teacher. After this we would meet to disucss her further treatment.

The tests showed no sign of dyslexia, but an accumulation of related spelling mistakes, suggesting that she had missed out on effective learning during her first years in school. Because of her age and the gaps in her education she began the third grade again the next fall, half a year after our initial contact with her.

After extensive psychiatric observation, including the use of sandbox, fingerpaint, and clay, I was able to confirm her father's assumption that Bluebird's learning disability was rooted in distinct emotional conflict. This had already resulted in serious problems in school, and I therefore arranged with her parents that she start a long-term once-a-week psychotherapy. I would brief her parents after half a year of therapy, and otherwise be in touch if need should be.

At the start of her first session, in September, Bluebird is pleasantly surprised to find that she is expected to paint. I offer her pencil and paper, crayons and poster colors and paint brushes in various sizes. She asks politely but eagerly what she is supposed to draw.

"Whatever you like," is my suggestion, "it doesn't have to be great art. The most important thing is that it's *your* picture, and not something you have seen elsewhere."[3] She chooses a pencil first, then crayons. Works eagerly. Her facial features reveal a deeply concentrated mind.

The central theme in her first picture, (Picture no. 1) is the tree and the bird flying from left to right. The tree appears first and has a solid trunk placed firmly on the ground and branches spreading out at the top. The outline of the tree is drawn in pencil, the trunk and branches are colored light brown with a crayon. The branches are studded with pale green leaves, and on the ground underneath the tree grow field flowers. I describe the pictorial content for her as I see it. I get the impression that the tree stands for a certain measure of growth, although it looks a bit windblown,[4] and say:

"Fine, something that's growing!"

Whereupon she draws the bird between the two mountains and the sun in two colours.[5]

"This is clearly *your* picture!"

She responds promptly by drawing a conventional cartoon-character in the shape of a rabbit, and looks at me teasingly.

"Good, you understand what I mean! — But what about the bird?"

She says,

"The bird flies to other countries, doesn't have to go to school!"[6]

"We'll have to do more of this!"

Bluebird obviously liked the idea and declared to her mother back in the waiting room that she wanted to come back and draw more!

The next session starts with "having it out with the teacher". (Picture no. 2). Bluebird herself calls the picture, "My world, last year," — last year meaning last school year. Her comments on the picture are:

"The teacher is hitting the thin air, I'm beating her with my closed fist."

The teacher (female) is in the center of the picture with a blue body, an ill-humoured mouth with lips sagging at the corners, and yellow, bristly hair. Bluebird is painted to the right, blue stripes in her hair, arms considerably elongated and "closed fists beating down on the teacher". Her best friend and the birds are helping her. Her friend is painted in a horizontal position to the right, [7] she too with a strikingly elongated arm.

"The principal is on the teacher's side!"

He is painted to the left with a gold crown on his head and a raised left hand, fingers spread out stiffly. The birds are circling over the combatants and are getting dangerously close to the principal's fingers.

"Who are those birds?" I ask.

"All my class-mates, they help me in the fight, pulling the principal's hair. The principal can't make a fist. He mustn't hit or the birds will bite him!"

Bluebird gets carried away, but refers only to the immediate situation, the school situation. From Bluebird's intense emotional involvement, which indicates that a compelling inner drive has forged this picture into existence, I get the impression that this is a multi-determined picture, consisting of several themes, with the themes extracted from more than one level of consciousness.[8] I comment on the most obvious element in the composition:

"It looks like you're getting plenty of support in the fight! But the picture is very complex, you need to make it clearer."

In her next session she paints *The Secret Lake* (Picture no. 3). A reddish-brown lake with a yellow center is the picture's main theme. Around the lake grow brown trees with blue, green, red, and violet leaves. Both before and after this picture she paints several "butterfly-pictures".[9] She is obviously concealing something. She is not able to offer any associations to the lake beyond the fact that it is "mysterious". This is, of course, significant in itself. We have a deal, however: I will tape pictures of special importance on a strip of paper that runs from ceiling to floor. We have started hanging them from the bottom. Every time we reach the ceiling, we will talk about what we have achieved. I now tell her that I consider *The Secret Lake* to be such a picture, and suggest that I hang it up.[10] She has time for a graphic comment before the session is over — a new version of the lake. It is painted in a darker shade of reddish-brown and a blue lady is reflected in the water. It strikes me later that the secret lake with the lady is intended to be a reflection of herself, that she is staging some sort of magic play.[11]

Next time, as I remind her of the mysterious picture from last time, she says:

"I just remembered something that I've seen!" And she paints *The Spring*. (Picture no. 4)

"It's a spring with very clear water that's coming from deep down in the ground. There are a lot of animals, fish and stuff like that down at the bottom, seaweed too — and a tall mountain."

She paints as she talks. Above the seascape she paints a bright sun and two birds flying towards the left. There is restless movement in the picture. She works rapidly as always when there is something that she needs to communicate, but does not want to put into words. She wants me to hang up the picture right away, and distracts me quickly and effectively by telling me a long story about her new class and how she wishes she was back in her old class!

Now I understand what her parents meant when they told me that she is difficult to manage. The process of transference is on. But what is she trying to avoid here?

On 1st November I remind her again about the mysteriousness in her lake-picture. She wants to paint something "funny and light", but it ends up "brown, black and heavy". (Picture no. 5) A large brown house with no windows or doors, but a chimney with thick, black smoke. Two birds are flying towards the left. Lately she has repeatedly included two birds in her pictures, and I have quietly assumed that they represent Bluebird and her sister. (Her sister is 2 years younger, socially mature, well adjusted, and does well in school. The parents have not mentioned sibling rivalry, only that Bluebird always insists on everything being "fair".)

It is obvious that something is in the air, but so far the birds haven't attacked each other. In the second picture this session (Picture no. 6) two girls are up in the mountains.

"It's windy and it's in the old days. They are playing 'Truant'. It's more exciting than going to school, and they can do more things. They don't need that much to survive, they can shoot an animal and sell the pelt."

"They are in the mountains?"

"Yes, but they don't want too many strangers to know who they are."

"You keep many fine secrets from me, too!" Above the biggest of the two girls, the blue bird is still flying towards the left.

In the next session we get *The Viking Spoil*. (Picture no. 7.)

"It is in a dream, like on the stage. I see boats, many different boats, viking-ships ...," she says, while painting in lustrous reddish-brown and yellow, first a church in flames (to the left), the steeple clearly with a phallic shape. Then a vaulted building to the right, and on the ground floor "a side-door, and two men are carrying out a chest, it is very heavy. They must get the things out."

Black smoke clouds the dramatic scene. A brown viking-ship appears between the church and the vaulted building, and vikings rush ashore. (Dirty-green lines). Way over to the right is a burning ship.

About the black smoke she says,

"It's *not* a mourning color, like before when people who were wearing black clothes, were in mourning."

The whole thing happens very quickly and before I get a chance to put down any cues, she is on to a new picture.

Her picture, *The Viking Spoil*, abounds with condensed symbolism. But the only thing I know for sure is: a phallus is on fire; treasure is stolen from the lower level of a femininely vaulted building, and the whole scene is produced "like a stage-show".

Besides the negative and educative comment about the black smoke, I did not get any more comments on this picture from Bluebird. The picture was produced while she was in a fantasizing, dreamy state of mind, and I regard it as a projection of pre-conscious and unconscious memory-fragments. The scene is displaced in time to "the old days", and the "actors" are disguised by an inner censoring agent. The picture is closely related to a dream where the main character is herself, and the main issue is fulfilment of infantile sexual wishes. [12]

Conservatively speaking, one might say that Bluebird's wish fulfilment as expressed here, censored, makes two interpretations[13] possible: either she wishes to be robbed herself or she wishes to be the person who steals the treasures. I read it this way: a destructive element (in the shape of a viking ship) forces itself between the masculine sex-symbol (disguised as a church steeple) and the feminine sex symbol (the vaulted house), and the main character, Bluebird, is disguised as a plundering viking. The fact that *two* men are carrying out the treasure may be due to the censoring agent. From general dream-interpretation theory we know that the main character always is the person who is dreaming. I therefore assume that Bluebird presented an infantile sexual wish of a destructive nature directed at her mother's body, overlaid by the oedipal wish to be her father's lover, and that her superego forced her to express fearfully that I need not mourn for her mother, even if she is robbed of her unique treasures, the contents of her uterus. ("it's *not* a mourning color"). I had at this point a firm but not yet documented impression that Bluebird was experiencing intense sibling rivalry and excessive aggression towards her internalized mother-figure.

Probably this picture describes Bluebird's relationship to both her father and sister in regard to her mother, and finally her relationship to me as a transference-figure.[14] I describe the pictorial content for her and get in response first a picture of a large "Africa-boat" that she wishes to travel on, and later a third version of the mysterious lake in the forest. Her censoring agent is clearly active, preventing further enlargement on the theme.

The next two sessions abound with diversionary efforts and playing around. I confront her with her resistance by pointing to the various ways she has disguised the real issues in her previous pictures.

"We need to do something about this. You can't create something new without overcoming the resistance in the material you are creating it from."

She does not really get started again until 29th November, this time with 11 pictures painted very quickly. The first of the pictures indicates the direction this theme is going to take (Picture no. 8): In from the right comes "a pipe that lets out dangerous fumes". To the left appears, sketchily, a "boot that smokes a pipe". (She has previously scolded me for smoking.) At the top left-hand corner she paints "a butterfly, a little weird". Then in the middle: "a sun that's shining". This gets painted over, obscured. On the ground are "happy colors, I'm thinking that it's summer with blue and purple flowers". To the right of the sun glides the blue bird, but now in a new and freer style.

In her next picture (Picture no. 9) she expands on the same theme. She puts it this way:

"It's the same picture, but later." (The pipe enters from the right again, and sprays a web of black paint all over the sheet.)

"The sun was destroyed. *(May be seen dimly as a yellow patch to the left).* The pipe is broken too, the bird is on the ground and the flowers are dead. The poison is being sprayed all over, that's why everyone is dead!"

I sum up the pictorial content and the expressive qualities, and as a reply I get a third picture that also describes the situation "after a while":

"It's almost all dark now." (The black paint covers almost the whole sheet.) Then she produces the same scene again:

"As soon as I paint it gets all black here! And the sheet is now all black."

She says:

"It's like when they bring the stage-curtain down and it's all over." I agree with her that this is what it looks like, but she corrects herself and says that it's really only time for a break! Another picture makes its way into existence with vivacious blue, green, red, brown and yellow stripes all over the sheet and she says:

"Black was the leader at first, but little by little the other colors took over." A long line of non-figurative pictures follow in bright colors where "flowers grow again and the sun returns." Finally she wants to paint "just one more picture":

"The blue and the green push away the black — it's not all beautiful, but not bad either!"

I have described this particular session thoroughly because the theme of *The Viking Spoil* is being worked through here and expanded on. The central theme is the penis-symbol, the pipe, that through its aggressive behaviour causes misery and death.

However, towards the end of the session, she manages to repair the destruction. Strong, healthy colors almost succeed in pushing the black, aggressive, retaliative element away, and when the session is over, she even indulges in a little joke and paints the word STOP, signifying the end of the session. The "O" develops into a stunned face with hair sticking up in the air. (Picture no. 10.)

In *The Viking Spoil* she appropriated her father's virility in the shape of his penis, assaulted the maternal capacity of her mother's uterus by destroying its content. In the picture of the deathly black penis we witness the retribution for such a gruesome deed: the sun doesn't shine anymore, the flowers die, even Bluebird falls to the ground. For the time being, all of this happens on the stage, so to speak. She has indicated briefly that I am a part of the play ("the boot smoking a pipe", the pipe also breaks). But the action has *nothing* to do with herself. In other words, the time is not ripe for any interpretation.

I continue to work with her resistance. The 26th session gives me a good opportunity to do this, and we are a little further on now. (Picture no. 11.)

She calls it *The Stage Curtain*.

"This curtain is closed, but a little open. And it *is* made to be opened." Beneath the curtain we see only the feet of numerous dancers. She herself is going to dance on the stage and the audience (she points to me) may watch. I tell her,

"The meaning of some things may be twofold. Here for instance I think that you want to open yourself up to me and not just hide." She responds by filling out a sheet of paper completely with pink, blue, and white paint, like a curtain, and says:

"This is the backdrop before the dancers arrive on the scene." Then she paints another picture that eventually gets all black. It depicts "some people dressed up like ghosts." Then comes a picture where the "good guy" (pink) chases the black and grey "bad guy" into jail. Then her brush performs a dance across a fresh sheet of paper; the "dance" finally ends up in an all pink sheet. I suggest that it may be a love-dance, and she nods and quickly paints two more pictures. The first one shows "a person who steals from another person and forgets that somebody stole from her before." In the last picture (grey-black) she ends up in jail.

"I think this means that you can get punished if you love someone. You have told me that it feels safe to hold your father's hand when you walk around town together and you worry that something bad has happened to mother. You have transferred this feeling of being safe to me now."[15]

In the next session I remind her of the dance scene from last time and she paints a picture where she is a rocket heading upwards to the left (Picture no. 12). She encounters me in the shape of a "magnifying glass that is going to show her the way and warn her about all the dangers that lurk about in space." The picture is sketchily done without any artistic concern and without conscious effort to cover up the content through "proper" drawing methods. I view the picture as a projection of her budding understanding of the psycho-analytical process and of her positive feelings towards father being transferred to me. I praise her:

"I think you gave a fine response to what we discussed last time."

When Bluebird returns after her Christmas vacation, I remind her of the rule about free association, with total discretion on my part. For an answer she picks up a large sheet of paper and paints *The Homing Pigeons* (Picture no. 13). First comes "something nice and free, not a jail". It turns into a tall blue mountain to the right. A thick, brown frame encases the mountain. Up the mountainside wander the pigeons, carrying mail. "No one can steal such mail, and this sky never gets clouded with bad weather." Eventually it becomes a tale of the pigeons she wishes for, but doesn't get. I tell her that the picture may mean two things at the same time: that one can talk freely in the therapy room without getting punished, and that she wants pigeons. I point to the free, blue mountain and the sky that never gets clouded and show her the connection: one can talk freely both there and here in this room.

"In the same way, there is a frame around the picture, as this room is confined by walls. Nothing gets out!" Bluebird gets thoughtful, but in the end the here-and-now takes over: she wants to save money and make a house for the pigeons.

In her next session she spontaneously paints a large blue bird (Picture no. 14) flying to the left. The bird covers almost the whole sheet and is painted in a clear, cobalt blue postercolor.[16] About the bird she says:

"It's a bird or a pigeon, it's really supposed to be white — invisible, in other words. It is before people existed. The bird wants to see other birds, other trees and other ways of life. It's windy but this bird can fly even when it gets really windy."

"I think this bird is a very important part of you. It wants to look into things that happened earlier in your life." She responds by painting a picture of a horse. (Picture no. 15) She thinks I know about it, it is a long time ago, also this from before there were people in the world, so she only made up what it was going to look like.

"It has a big, black tail, spotted like a ... whatever, and you see its shadow behind it."

"I think there are two horses, father and I, that almost overlap."

She is already into her next picture. (Picture no. 16) We can dimly see a black figure painted over with blue lines and dots. A little yellow paint blends in with the blue. Her running commentary:

"Two black arms, it's turning into a black figure, a Chinese? It looks a little weird."

"I wonder what the blue is?"

"It's only rain, and the yellow is there because the sun is shining — a little!"

The picture is titled *A black Chinese who walks behind a painting*. I tell her I think it is her mother whom she is angry with and loves, (she has described the person as "she"). I also describe the black arms, all of the black figure for her.

"But at the same time you let the sun shine through!" Bluebird nods in consent and paints the last picture this session. She calls it *A Planet*. The picture seems like a real fantasia, incomprehensible — for the time being ... (see *The Planet-Car Driver* which arrives later.)

To sum it up, we now have a large picture of an exploring blue bird, herself. We have a double portrait of father and me — the two horses. And we have a portrait of a black mother-figure, where "the sun is shining through". What happened to her sister?

On 24th January a large yellow lion enters the scene (Picture no. 17). She says that the lion is the boss, and that it represents herself.[17]

"This is the fun thing about fairy-tales, you can change the order of things. That's why I'm the boss here!" Above the lion is her own birthday cake with 10 candles. Behind the lion comes a little rabbit "which thinks IT is the boss."

"The bunny is really a lady-lion, and since she isn't the strongest, she doesn't get to decide."

Bluebird tells me about a girl in her class "who is dumb because she thinks she is the strongest". I think Bluebird is moving about on several levels now — this picture seems to represent her relationship to her friend and her sister, as well as her mother.

"I'm beginning to think that the bunny mostly means your sister!" She responds with the second picture that session which is *A horse with a long-short mane*. (Picture no. 18)

"It's a stupid horse."

"Who does the long-short hair remind you of?" First she gives me the name of a girl in her class, then the former teacher. Finally she mentions her sister who recently cut her hair herself and was told off because it was uneven. Quickly she paints another picture which she hands me right away (Picture no. 19) as if it is burning her fingers. It shows "that stupid horse again" (to the right). To the left she has painted an enormous, yellow mouth with rows of sharp brown teeth.

"First you disguise your sister as a friend, then as your former teacher, just so I won't recognise her. Now I understand why: those yellow jaws don't look nice!" She does not answer, but draws another picture (Picture no. 20). Here comes the lion again. This time with black teeth and a "long blood-dripping tongue" hanging out.

"It has red, flashing eyes and is very angry."

"Blood-thirsty too?" She pulls back a little:

"The blood is there to scare people, it isn't real."

"I think you were really mad at your baby-sister."

The lion enters again, in a new drawing. This time with its tail sticking up. (Picture no. 21) I am curious about that tail, and question her about it, but get for an answer:

"It's bad (*the lion*), and happy to have someone on its team. It is as strong as I am, and has been here all the time." I tell her that I think she feels both bad and wicked, but relieved to have me with her. Bluebird nods in consent, but adds:

"... cut the mane for mom's sake."

This is said in a low voice, like an afterthought, not a direct communication.

Next time she paints *An Ugly Man*. (Picture no. 22) Tells me that this is art, makes another one on the same sheet, to the left.

"Who does this remind you of?"

"The stupid principal."

"And perhaps someone else?"

She is already on to the next picture. (Picture no. 23) I think it resembles a mask and tell her.

"No, it's the same man, only he's painted himself." And she paints still another face (Picture no. 24), while she tells me that "he thinks he's good-looking, but I think he's just stupid."

"It looks like you envy something that man has." She responds by painting with four brushes simultaneously *A Stupid Pump*. (Picture no. 25)

I suggest that it looks like a penis and point to the previous pictures of the principal, father and myself.

"Perhaps you envy all of us? And perhaps you wish you had a penis yourself?"

In her next session I do not even have to remind her of her previous theme. She paints *The Innocent Chewing Gum* (Picture no. 26). First she paints, in the center, a white chewing gum, then to the right, "something yummy, you haven't seen the like of it — oh, yes, you can buy it in paper bags, but I didn't get one." She points to various sweets to the right. To the left she paints "a candy cane, very special, you can only buy it in Denmark and America." It is painted in red, and above it she paints a lollipop, (in Norwegian: "love-on-a-stick"), below several "baby-chewing gums", and finally some J-shaped "noses" over the white chewing gum. I have interpreted some of this along the way and relate it to her:

"The white chewing gum is the innocent Bluebird who hasn't done anything wrong, the candy to the left is mommy-stuff, 'there's nothing like it'. To the right daddy-goodies, like a penis. And above these you have 'love-on-a-stick'. I think you love daddy very much. Finally you made two nose-things. I think these also have something to do with men. It looks like you are showing me again that you wish you had a penis."

Bluebird seems distracted and draws Picture no. 27. She says apologetically:

"I was just thinking about something." The picture shows a phallus-shaped object that is floating around inside a cloud. When she has finished drawing, she pulls from her pocket a multicolored pen. I imagine that her wishful thinking and the pen which is real thus merge and become one thing in her mind.

"Did daddy give that to you?"

"Yes, on the Seventeenth of May." (Independence Day in Norway.) She makes a quick sketch, *A hand stealing something — nobody knows what it is*". (Picture no. 28) Then: *The Green Chemicals* (Picture no. 29), shaped like "a green bomb, and it's really not dangerous!" Immediately above the bomb I find myself floating around in the shape of a "blue-red" cloud. The new teacher is also included in this drama, but she escapes by running out of the house. Bluebird is hesitant to make further comments, and I provoke her a little:

"Your stream of thought runs continuously. When you don't talk, it is perhaps because you are angry with me?" Upon which she paints, with ferocious speed, *The Planet-Car Driver and the Deadly Bomb*, (Picture no. 30). The picture is painted in a sharp green color, deadly green, so to speak. Inside a cloud a planet-car driver races along a vertical and a horizontal track. Underneath lies "a deadly bomb, in fact", inside a green box. She says:

"The planet-car driver gets really scared, hurt, but not dead — he will have a very poor life."

"To steal my penis is also to hurt me and then I won't have a very good life," is my comment.

Bluebird, however, is on to another sketch, *A woman's face floats in a cloud of green chemicals* (Picture no. 31). It is supposed to represent Bluebird's former teacher who has inhaled the fumes from some of the chemicals from the bomb.

"The chemicals make it so her brain won't think so well!"[18] And she adds, to be on the safe side:

"The chemicals are my own invention. It is an invention that helps me not to get sick. Actually, this is a picture of me. But that's a secret. No bad people are supposed to know about me, only the good ones," she says in a magical, self-assured way.[19]

She paints another sketch of *A baldheaded man* (She has

previously teased me about being bald) *with disgusting eyes, who is very mean*. (Picture no. 32).

"He makes bombs and kidnaps people, I call him The Bald One. That's a good name for him. He has lots of helpers, and a gun too."

"Can you draw him without a mask?" Whereupon she draws a black head (Picture no. 33). Sole comment:

"Can't remember exactly."

It is at this point I realize that Bluebird's pictures have become too personal to hang on the wall, and I suggest that we keep them in the closet. We have reached a critical stage. Her resistance is becoming more intense. She is continuously finding new ways to camouflage her messages.

In her next session she copies something from the newspaper padding on the table where she is painting. Gradually she develops "a secret language". She paints several pictures with cryptic ciphers. Discovers also that "white is a good color". With it she can not only make them lighter, she can also make them invisible. I support her inventiveness, but not the destructive direction it is taking here. She understands the situation and paints a horizontal line across the middle of the sheet: one one side is Bluebird camouflaging everything with white paint; on the other myself, taking down notes! (Picture no. 34). It is in this session that she invents the cover-up term KLUZ (Picture no. 35)[20].

Finally she paints an orange bonfire where she symbollically burns all the smear (kluz) (Picture no. 36). Inscribed on the bonfire is a large red and a large black "X", signifying that both what I say and what she paints is false.

"It looks like you are getting tired both of your own diversionary KLUZ and of the fact that I am constantly reminding you that it's holding you back."[21]

She paints 13 pictures the next time. It is impossible to relate all of them. The first one is simply a large green apple, (Picture no. 37) with a black stem and blossom part, naturalistic and pretty.

"It's an ordinary apple." While painting another one in red, she says:

"I'm just green. The red one is my sister."

"I thought you were green with envy?"

"I thought envy was black."

"Okay, so you've been black with envy, just like that black stem. Maybe it was a long time ago, and may be it was especially because she took mommy from you. This is why the stem is still black." She smiles while she paints a big fat man who is "very dumb or very kind" (picture no 38).

"I think that stupid-kind man is me telling you that you were black with envy of your sister!" She laughs and paints a large house in that particular "bluebird-blue" that she likes so much (Picture no. 39). The next picture turns into a palette consisting of the colors she normally uses in the sessions.

"There is something good that wants to help me." Then follows something vague in green that quickly gets painted over with blue. I say:

"It looks like the blue, good, kind paint wins."[22]

She continues on another sheet. Starts with my climbing plant which she paints in bluebird blue (Picture no. 40). After a while she says,

"It's ended up looking like a stove, and it's lit — you can see the stove is smoking. But blue plants are growing out of it, too."

"I think you are grateful for coming here." She paints "a lady without a head, a skeleton," and another, smaller figure who "kicks the skeleton". (Picture no. 41).

"But it looks like you left something out?" Instead of answering she quickly sketches my pants leg and shoe and asks:

"What are you going to use my pictures for?"

"I'm going to make a book out of them."

"I'll have to make a good drawing then! Will people be able to buy that book?"

"Yes."

"Okay, then I'll buy it!" And she paints a "giant forest" (picture no. 42), thousands of trees grow here, so tall you can't see the top, and here is me": a little blue girl in a purple skirt.

"It turned into a little girl between tall trees . . ."

"I'll give you more," she says and paints a self-portrait:

"A weird person with her head covered up and hair that's sticking up because I rubbed it with 'kluz'."

"Perhaps you are also a little afraid of getting your pictures in a book?" Whereupon she sketches *A girl dancing happily to the right, and on her head a hat that's a commercial for my sister* (Picture no. 43). On leaving the room after this session, she says:

"Now that stupid man has turned into a very nice man!"

The crisis is over, her relationship to me has taken a turn for the better. I have refrained from commenting on her deadly fight with the "lady-skeleton".

From now on, new issues will be introduced, to be pursued or let go; and issues that I thought were resolved, will reappear with renewed force, in fresh and stunning pictorial language.

Thus in her next session too (Picture no. 44) a purple dress features. Bluebird paints from the bottom up, first a large, wide skirt. She smiles a cryptic smile. Next comes the bodice, then sleeves in the same color, decorated with pink stripes. The face is painted brown, the hair black and rich, with bows in it.

"At first it was going to be me as a little girl, but then it turned into a lady-singer on TV." I sense that she is communicating something about the problems of being in therapy.

"You have painted a lot from a long time ago, from when you were little. But you're a big girl now, ten years old. This is what happens when you are in therapy, you become both big and little at the same time. Perhaps you noticed this when you were going to paint this girl?" She asks for a fresh sheet and paints a dense green forest with snow on the ground and ski-tracks. (Picture no. 45).

"You can't see the tracks up close, only from a distance." She goes on to associate to a skiing trip with daddy the day before and paints a large yellow sun that fills up almost the whole of the next sheet of paper.

"I think you were daddy's sweetheart?" She rushes to say that "the lady doesn't belong in the forest."

"What lady?"

"The lady singer."

"I think you want to be alone with daddy without mommy." She paints the palette again (Picture no. 46). This time the dots of paint are arranged in the shape of a house. A cat is peeking out of one of the windows:

"It fooled you! It's teasing you!" she says.

"I think YOU're teasing me!" She nods, grabs an earlier kluz-drawing and covers the lady singer with it.

I produce the palette-picture next time she comes and as a response I get Picture no. 47. It starts with a "double figure" in blue in the middle of the sheet. The two figures are then combined to form a sweater. Beneath the sweater she paints a purple skirt, then hands, feet, face and "thick, black hair that's blowing in the wind."

"It looks like a girl I drew before, not here, at home."

"Perhaps it looks like you?"

"No, it's not me."

"The leaves are blowing off the trees, is it in the fall?"

"No, not fall, it's just windy."

Quickly she paints a red sun above the tree. I say:

"It started out like a dream-picture, then it became a more ordinary picture, the kind you paint at home?" She nods and says.

"I do not have black hair," whereupon she quickly starts painting a more abstract, symbolic picture (Picture no. 48). I call it *Bluebird between Two Suns*, and she says,

"There are two suns and a blue storm."

"You're out in the storm, then. I guess that means you are having a tough time. Perhaps I have become more like mommy than daddy to you?"[23]

She paints a third picture (picture no. 49), where she has kept the red sun, "the yellow has turned into a half moon", and in the middle wanders a little girl on a round, blue globe. She says the figure is herself and that "she is quite near the sun." The black that surrounds her is "because it's in outer space, and the little figure is both sad and happy."

The symbolic content is extremely condensed.

"In outer space? I think it's in this room." Quickly she paints two kluz-pictures in black, the one is placed on top of the first picture; the other covers the third picture. Only the abstract picture is left uncovered. I ask whether she has dreamed anything that can clarify this theme. She tells me a dream she had two days ago after seeing a film on TV about poor children in Asia.

"I was on an airplane, someone else was steering, no one else dared because it made a lot of turns. There were two black birds, each one in a cage, on both sides. They couldn't see each other. The plane went awfully fast, it was a beautiful place — Africa — the biggest country in the world, large houses, and children on the garbage heaps."

"Can you paint the part about the two birds?" She paints a black bird behind bars" (Picture no. 50).

"The bird was looking out of the cage, I saw its eyes through the bars." It turned into a small, knotted sketch.

"And there were cloth-walls on both sides, could have fallen out, it was great fun, I was on the floor, lifted up the cloth-wall, and there to the right, someone was steering. We were on our way back from Africa, couldn't find Mommy, a lady was speaking a foreign language, I couldn't understand her. Mommy was in Africa, but at the same time she wasn't."

"What about the cloth walls?"

"They were fluttering in the wind, we could have a good look, the cloth walls were red."

"Did the plane make that many loops?"

"It made loops the whole time."

Probably this picture is about having witnessed a sexual act, but so far I have not understood everything concerning the mother's part in it.

"What about Mommy who was there and was not there?"

"There were two ladies there, one had grey hair, and one had black hair. Mommy has black hair."

The session is over, I do not have time to pursue this theme.[24]

Her first picture in the next session depicts *A bluish-purple island rising from a black ocean* (Picture no. 51). The sun is large and red, it is setting. Her own association to the picture is at first that it is "a painting';', but then she retracts and says that it is *her* picture. I interpret it this way myself. She has no further comments, however, and her subsequent efforts become investigations into the use of colors. The colors and shapes suggest that the picture is yet another picture of her mother.[25]

At the beginning of the next session I inform Bluebird that I have recently had a conversation with her parents, where we agreed to continue the therapy "and that the goal now is to become an even better explorer". I also inform her that we have eight sessions left before we have to take a break for four months, since I will be going away. She tells me eagerly about her own trip — she is visiting relatives alone for a whole month. During the conversation she is painting a picture (Picture no. 52). It depicts *Two Islands in the Ocean*, is done in thick paint of her favorite blue color and resembles two raised breasts. To the right: "running water". I take the opportunity to ask her to paint Mommy. The result is one of her typical sketches that are not premeditated (Picture no. 53). The picture is rendered in blue. In the center is Mommy with her left arm raised, ready to hit. Later this is changed to depict her mother balancing a tray of buns. In her right hand she is holding a travelling bag. To the right Bluebird draws herself, to the left her sister, flinging out an elongated hand to pull Bluebird's hair. About the picture as a whole, she says that she is finally going to travel on her own! I tell her that the picture is very condensed and that she and Mommy have changed places in it — I think that the figure in the center is Bluebird with a travelling bag and her arm raised.

"You are angry with Mommy but at the same time you love her."

"Mommy doesn't make buns."

"Exactly! But now it's your turn to leave her! Too bad for your sister, she is in a bad mood, she's angry and she is crying!" I point to the expression on her sister's face and the elongated arm. Excited and proud, Bluebird spends the rest of the session telling me about the trip and the camera Daddy is going to let her borrow.

The next time she comes I suggest that she use crayons, thinking that liquid paint as a medium may elicit stronger emotions at this stage than she can handle.[26] I remind her of her latest picture of Mommy. We go through the content of it; because of the Easter holidays two weeks have passed since she painted it.

Her first drawing is of *A little Easter chicken on a green lawn* (Picture no. 54). Next to it appears a mother hen, which is then changed into a rooster.[27] To the right a pencil-shaped man tipping his hat — the man is bald. Beneath the grass she draws a lion with a raised tail and an open mouth with two rows of sharp teeth.

"It was supposed to be a lion," she says and wants to put it away.

"I think it looks scary, like it wants to bite!"

She then picks up a theme from three sessions back about the moon, the planet earth and the sun. She paints a blue-green globe in the middle, the earth. Above is a large red sun and in the upper left-hand corner a small yellow moon. Many small planets follow (Picture no. 55). I get the impression that this is a naturalistic picture of space and interpret it as a flight from the aggressive lion, and tell her so. She continues on a fresh sheet, a small house and an odd, segmented road that leads to the house. The road ends up in a cul-de-sac (Picture no. 56). She says that the picture was "a mistake", and draws a corrected version on the back of the sheet (Picture no. 57). The house is larger now, the road more winding, but it still has no outlet. This drawing is also "a mistake", she says, whereupon she produces an entirely new version. Here, in pencil, she draws a human figure. The right leg she calls "the runner"; the body becomes "a tree", (Picture no. 58). The tree has "an entrance to a cave" below, which is marked in red like "the runner's" foot. A tunnel with a lit candle winds its way up towards the cave, which is square and placed in the abdominal area. The "body" has no head, but two branch-like arms. Inside the square which she calls "the cave" is a figure.

"Call it a bunny," she says.

"I think it looks like a human head with two arms — could it be a baby in the mother's uterus?"

She responds by drawing "a water-fall" on the back of the sheet. The water-fall is red (Picture no. 59). Behind the water-fall is a cliff with a round cave in it, and a tunnel leads from the cave to "a niche with food". These drawings are executed in a hurry, whereupon Bluebird turns to leafing through the newspaper padding on the table and coloring photos in the newspaper.

I assume that she has created another version of *The Viking Spoil*, on a deeper level, and that it confirms my interpretation.[28]

The next time she comes, she is very secretive, and the session is spent experimenting with paint on a wet sheet. She concentrates on making one color run into another, and says:

"I didn't know I could control it so well."

All the pictures are destroyed — first a clown, then a portrait of me, a mask and a crocodile. Also a portrait of her sister is lost in the same manner. I am not pleased with the way this technique destroys her pictures, and I tell her so.

Since it is getting close to the time of my going away, I plan to work through old issues in the remaining six sessions.

In her next session she tells me about her own trip and on a sheet of paper she renders "the most dangerous thing that can happen" — but black paint gradually covers all of it. She picks up the theme on a fresh sheet. This picture is kept in black with blue stripes and patches of red:

"It's something to do with Mom-Mom's disease and blue patches — she died when Mommy was 14 years old. I started thinking about it while I was painting in black."

It reminds her of red wine pouring out of a tank (— an accident she has seen on TV).

"I think that the most dangerous thing that can happen has to do with Mommy and death," is my suggestion. "But we have to look at that next time, because the session is over."

The next time she starts out painting green grass at the bottom of the sheet, and I ask her what she is thinking about.

"Nothing."

"I don't believe that, because people think the whole time."

She picks up another sheet, "to practise". It turns into a light blue looped line. She tries again on a fresh sheet. This time "a sliding board with a swimming pool" appears, with a big, bright sun in the background (Picture no. 60).

"You have painted this beautiful sun many times before in pictures about Daddy." She wants a fresh sheet and paints a bell-shaped, purple hat, (that is, I'm supposed to think it is a hat — she smiles teasingly). It ends up like a frowning "witch" (Picture no. 61).

"What does this remind you of?"

"Mommy."

The next picture is in brown and black paint. First she paints again "a brown hat" that is not a hat, then the rest of a body in brown with black trousers and black hair.

"Does this remind you of anybody?"

"No."

She grabs a new sheet of paper and paints with ferocious speed a pasquinade of her sister in purple (Picture no. 62).

"She always wants pink, because she loves pink." She sounds contemptuous. "I should have painted something in pink, but I couldn't."

"Give it a try!"

She grabs a sheet and furiously beats at the sheet with her

brush. Purple paint is splashed all over the sheet, and gets covered with brown paint. She seems to have gotten it all out and says apologetically:

"I just made a mistake, and then I 'kluz'ed' it out, so now I'm finished with it."

"Oh, really? I've never seen you this angry!"

Next session, I remind her of the sliding board and Daddy, the witch and Mommy, her furious attack on her sister. She draws a triangle, a square and a circle. I describe these shapes as "angular and angry", "round and soft". She turns her sheet over and paints *The Truck-Drivings* (Picture no. 63). In the center of the sheet a truck races up a bumpy hill. It is light blue. Behind it a red car is also speeding up the hill. On a different road, to the right, climbs another truck painted in the purple color that is her sister's. Down in the left-hand corner is "something nice in a sort of cradle", above it "a fat guy". Finally, in the upper left-hand corner, a "sunshine car". I tell her that the picture is getting clear now:

"First there's you and Daddy, in a close race, then your sister, on her own, then, you and I, down in the left-hand corner — you in the cradle, all snug and comfortable, I, a 'fatso' in green. Above it all — well, what do you mean by 'sunshine car'?"

Bluebird responds with a new picture (Picture no. 64).

"It's a 'make-believe' picture."

"A picture that you have inside you?"

First comes "a bent rod" in red, then, "blue foot-prints from a spider near the tip of the rod."

"Spiders mean happiness if you don't kill them," she says.

To the right she paints a few stars.

"Show me even more clearly!"

In her next picture she rolls out the paint with the handle of the brush.

"It feels g-o-o-d making all these lines!"

She makes a squeaking sound by scratching the paper with the handle of the brush.

"Listen!"

"What does the spider remind you of?"

"The car — and that squeaking sound reminds me of the engine."

"You also said that spiders mean happiness — if nobody kills them."

Another sheet of paper. Broad strokes of the brush spread purple paint across the sheet.

"I was just going to catch up with the polka-dots!"

"What polka-dots?"

She picks up another sheet and repeats the purple smear.

"Right now I'm not thinking about anything!"

She makes another version of the smear, in cerulean blue, and says:

"I don't want you to know what it is, because I don't know what it's going to be!"

On another sheet of paper the polka-dots become parked cars.

"It looks like you want to make a full stop here!"

In the remaining sessions I let her try some acrylic paint which her mother has agreed to let her use at home when I go away. Picture no. 65 is one of these pictures. She spends a lot of time on this painting and it turns into a landscape with a tall tree in the center, a large yellow sun, green grass with blue and red flowers. In the foreground a deep, blue, winding river. Finally, near the sun, she paints "a white dove!" Works hard at it, fails, and the dove becomes "a white cloud" instead. I remind her of the fact that the big blue bird (Picture no. 14) "should actually have been a white dove", that is, invisible.

The remaining part of the therapy may prove to be the most demanding. At this point in the therapy, however, the parents are pleased with Bluebird's progress, and she is also doing better in school.

Notes to Narrative

1. i.e. the regional psychiatric out-patient clinic for children and adolescents.
2. "Dyslexia" as used here refers to a reading/writing disability due to a developmental disorder or an organic dysfunction of the brain.
3. I inform the children that "free" picture production is the No. 1 rule.

4. Wind is a recurrent theme in her pictures, symbolizing external problems/inner conflicts, see Picture no. 14: "The blue bird that can fly even when it gets very windy."
5. It appears later that the sun in two colors symbolizes the love/hate relationship to her internalized mother. (See note no. 5, Introduction.) The yellow sun clearly symbolizes her internalized father.
6. The bird clearly represents something in herself: a tendency to run away from problems through fantasizing and regression. ("flies to other countries, doesn't go to school"). The tree probably represents a part of her too, the ambitious, strong, stubborn, and righteous part of her. It has not been confirmed yet in this therapy, but generally trees represent ego-supporting forces. The tree is the first object she draws here, and she places it in the center of the sheet — details that are repeated in later pictures.

   The first picture is of special interest in that it often contains several of the main issues — issues which will reappear later in the therapy.
7. In children's drawings elongated arms express strength. Another detail which departs from a naturalistic presentation of the scene is the fact that one person (her friend) is presented in a horizontal position. This is done to increase the pictorial impact of the attack.
8. The level of consciousness which the various emotional issues originate from could be the following: relationship to female teacher — conscious, disguising relationship to mother — near-conscious, disguising relationship to therapist — unconscious, relationship to male principal — conscious, disguising relationship to father — near-conscious, disguising relationship to therapist — unconscious.
9. A "Butterfly-picture" is produced by pouring a little paint in the center of the sheet, folding the sheet together and squeezing out the paint thoroughly. This is a common nursery-school activity. The resulting symmetrical designs resemble Rorschach-plates. (Projective psychological test developed by Dr. Rorschach.) Bluebird makes use of such pictures here to avoid the real issues — and this tendency serves the same purpose as, and intensifies, her habit of fantasizing.

10. The purpose of this deal was to emphasize pictures that needed to be worked through. Our deal about summing up was a reminder that the therapy was not perpetual. This deal was later changed when the pictures assumed a more private character. From then on all pictures were kept in a closet, but we continued to call attention to the more significant ones.
11. The magical form which her defense assumes as time goes by should be viewed with regard to the sub-paranoid misconceptions that are revealed as she works through her relationship to her internalized mother.
12. Sigmund Freud in *Traumdeutung*, (1900), ("Drommetydning", II, Cappelen, Oslo 1985, p. 257,) states that the central part of a dream is the satisfaction of wishes (translated from the Norwegian): "It is the satisfaction of wishes that has caused us to divide dreams into two groups. We have seen dreams that presented themselves quite openly as satisfaction of wishes, and others where the satisfaction of wishes was unrecognizable and often disguised by various means. In the latter we saw the achievements of the dream censor ... the strength of the wish impulse equals that of infantilism ... the hyperamnesia of the dream and its access to childhood material have become the corner stone of our doctrine; in our dream theory we have ascribed the role of primus motor of dream-making to the wish of the infantile ..."
13. At this time no interpretation was given. I regarded this stage as "a time to understand" and not as "a moment to conclude". (Lacan, 1936.)
14. This condensed situation is like a fugue for four voices where one voice merges with another, in an orderly fashion, yet freely and playfully, until all the voices join in in a counterpoint synthesis — not unlike the complicated inner dream work that precedes the remembered dream.
15. One of the reasons why her parents consulted us was Bluebird's phobic worry that something like bag-snatching should happen to her mother. The bag-snatching is probably disguising her unconscious wish to appropriate the contents of the womb of her internalized mother-image.

16. In her first picture the bird is less conspicuous; here it takes up almost all the space. If we carry this comparison further, we see initially a multicolored bird flying towards the right in a windswept landscape, between two tall mountains and a sun in two colors. This time an oversize, monocrome bird is flying to the left, and this bird is projected at a time when she finds herself in a therapeutically controlled, regressive state. Several researchers of this subject (e.g. Annelise Bude, see list of references) have previously noted that in a graphic projection of unconscious material the direction right to left means that one is turning to the unconscious, whereas turning to the right means turning to the conscious, the future, the progressive.
    I think the bird is an expression of her main diversionary manoeuvre — her tendency to run away from reality, from difficulties and conflicts. But this very tendency has been made a creative resource in the course of the therapy.
17. I believe this is the first time she spontaneously gives a part in the act to herself; she assures me, however, in her next sentence, that this is only a fairy-tale!
18. In all probability she has overheard some talk of possible brain damage in connection with discussions about dyslexia.
19. See note no. 11.
20. The term KLUZ is derived from a TV-program for young people "KLUZZ", and was prompted by my pointing to her diversionary manoeuvers — "avverge-kluss" meaning "diversionary mess".
21. My impression is that the righteousness has to do with a fundamental authority complex.
22. The blue color represents here the positive aspect of the father-transference situation, but on the verge of changing into representing the negative aspect of the mother-transference as it is disclosed in the fight with the lady skeleton later in this session. She associates the therapist with the same blue color.
23. A sign that the transference situation is shifting to a mother-transference is to be found in the episode where she kicks "the lady skeleton" (Picture no. 41) shortly after I have said: "I think you like coming here?"

24. I tried to have her paint associations to other parts of the dream, but we only had time for "the bird's cage."
25. The bluish-purple island could symbolize the new, positive image of inner mother; the previous one was characterized by the color black — see *"black ocean", "the black Chinese walking behind a painting"*, Picture no. 15.
26. I think that she may attack mother right now while a positive mother-image is emerging.
27. "The mother hen is changed into rooster": A theoretical understanding of what this projected image represents at this stage is given by Melanie Klein (*Contributions* ..., p. 208):

"I ... hold that the genital development of the woman finds its completion in the successful displacement of oral libido on to the genital — my results lead me to believe that this displacement begins with the first stirrings of the genital impulses and that the oral, receptive aim of the genitals exercises a determining influence in the girl's *turning to the father* ... "
p. 209: "— envy and hatred of the mother who possesses the father's penis seem, at the period when these first Oedipus impulses are stirring, to be a further motive for the little girl's *turning to the father* ... "
Bluebird returns to the attack on her mother-image in the archaic pictures, nos. 58 and 59. In the Kleinian way of thinking one could say that it is now possible for her to turn to her first love-object, mother.

28. The central theme in these pictures is the archaic uterine symbol. (See "Introduction", Archaic uterine symbols.)

DISCUSSION

DIAGNOSTIC

The explorations of Bluebird's character and personality all point towards distinct neurotic fixations of a compulsive nature. There are no signs of organic disorder. Special education tests reveal an exceptional capacity for symbolizing, but she achieves a low score on all tests involving learned skills.

Her main symptoms are her learning disability and her compulsive, regressive habit of fabulizing. Gradually certain subparanoid traits are revealed, characterized by an inclination to protect herself through a "magic" defense mechanism. No signs of a faulty perception of reality could be detected.

Her neurotic fixation is mainly rooted in the oral- and anal-sadistic psycho-sexual development phases, see the attack on her sister, Picture no. 19. She is fixated in an ambivalent, destructive conflict in her relationship to an internalized mother image (see Pictures no. 16, 41 and 51.) Accordingly the resolution of the oedipal conflict is delayed (see Pictures 7 – 10). Her sibling conflict is of a destructive nature and is closely related to her conflict with mother. Her learning disability is maintained and compounded by her strong inclination to fantasize, but its roots can also be traced back to her unresolved epistemophilic conflicts at the oral/anal-sadistic stage (see Picture no. 58 and 59).

Her resources are, besides her intellectual capacity, her remarkable gift for creative thinking which is revealed through her habit of fantasizing.

It seems reasonable to tie up her identification with the bird with her ambivalent relationship to her mother. An ambivalent conflict of such a destructive nature will readily evoke sub-paranoid or paranoid ideas, and such are often represented by the same symbol — birds. The sub-paranoid traits and the magic defence mechanism were uncovered during the treatment of her relationship to her internal mother image.

We observe that the bird symbolizes two contradictory elements. On the one hand there is a tendency to run away, fantasize, and regress. On the other hand, there is the tendency to explore, inquire, and develop. The large blue bird mostly represents the regressive element, whereas the smaller, multicolored bird represents the progressive element. Thus one might say that the bird is a symbolic expression of the main conflict in her psyche.

THERAPEUTIC GOAL

My main task is to attempt to reduce this ambivalence to her mother through a transference relationship with the therapist and to help her gain, through experience, the realization that her regressive pattern is no longer adequate. The balance between "the evil" and "the good" mother image will thus be altered so that the heavy side of the scale is no longer represented by the loathed, frightening, black mother symbols which we have seen in so many of her pictures, but by fresh symbols representing a person who can be expected to be present (see *The Dream of Africa*, Picture no. 50), who is supportive and accepting both in good times and bad. The ideal may be described as a "Good Enough Mother" (Winnicott, 1949), an internalized mother image whose main characteristic is positive.

Such a transference was in progress before the preliminary break in therapy; what remains to be achieved now is a firmer establishment and working through of the conflict through the transference situation.

The issue of sibling rivalry has been focused on several times and has been worked through. Its deepest roots are to be found in her relationship to her mother. This is true of the oedipal conflict as well. As far as the relationship to her father is concerned, some work remains to be done on problems related to the question of authority — revealed through Bluebird's righteousness. It is reasonable to assume that this tendency is tied to her father image only to a certain extent and that, in this respect too, improvement can be expected when the oral/anal-sadistic conflict has been more thoroughly worked through.

THERAPEUTIC METHOD

Art interpreting therapy, with its challenge to free picture production, might have the effect of intensifying Bluebird's compulsive habit of fabulizing. On the other hand, her gift for fabulizing is an important resource, and might, when employed in a controlled regressive therapy situation, serve to increase the beneficial effect of such treatment.

It has been necessary to restrict her fantasizing at times, for instance by encouraging verbal explanations or by directly challenging her to go through a certain picture with me one more time.

There have been few consciously designed pictures in this

therapy — even the early *Having it out with the teacher* (Picture no. 2) encompassed material from several layers of consciousness.

The Viking Spoil (Picture no. 7) was a typical pre-conscious, complex composition with great potential for therapeutic intervention. *The Truck Driver* (Picture no. 63) is another, similar example, showing how the pictorial language allows her to include her relationship to father, sister, and me in a quick, condensed composition.

Many sketchy pictures like *The Planet Car Driver*, Picture no. 30, *The Girl who's kicking a Skeleton*, Picture no. 41, *The Black Head*, Picture no. 33, and *The Spider and the red Stick*, Picture no. 64, indicate that the method evokes dream wishes in an unambiguous and emotional manner.

Projection of unconscious material as it appears in the pictures with the archaic uterine-symbols, (Pictures no. 58 and 59), reveals id-impulses and derivatives of these, here of an epistemophilic nature. The mother symbol, Picture no. 51, and the breast symbols, Picture no. 52, reveal a new image of mother in *status nascendi*.

The crucial question in evaluating the effectiveness of the method is whether the negative transference has been successful. Picture no. 30, *The Planet Car Driver*, Picture no. 32, *The Bald-headed man with disgusting Eyes*, and Picture no. 33, *The Black Head*, are examples indicating that such is the case.

2   Rocket

NARRATIVE

Rocket was 8 years old when his parents consulted us. They did so because the relationship between the boy and his mother had become "almost intolerable". He constantly attacked her both verbally and physically and his mother "had actually begun to worry what she might do to him."

The relationship between the boy and his father was less marred by conflict, but the father was aware of his wife's predicament.

Both parents felt that Rocket's motor coordination was immature, and that he was ungainly and slow. He was in the second half of his first school year. The home-room teacher shared his parents' view of him. He had problems reading and writing. He had not had his intellectual functioning tested, but he had one individual lesson a week of remedial reading instruction.

His sister was 3 years younger. She was bright and mature for her age. There were "signs of sibling rivalry," but the parents "had the situation well under control."

Play observation indicated that his problems were particularly related to a destructive, conflictive relationship to an internal mother-figure, and that he was belatedly experiencing an oedipal conflict together with intense sibling rivalry.

He functioned well intellectually, but his vocabulary was rather limited, with a poorly developed capacity for abstract thinking.

He displayed poor motor coordination, and also had symptoms indicating impaired eye-hand coordination. I recommended testing of cognitive functioning and, if necessary, more remedial tutoring.

The treatment started out as play therapy, 1 session a week, and lasted for half a year with 24 sessions altogether. His attempts to express his internal conflicts in the sandbox were laborious. His development was impeded by his inclination to think in concrete terms, and by a limited vocabulary.

It was obvious that sand, water, and traditional toys were unsuitable means of communication for him — he took a long time planning and working through the various sequences. I therefore suggested art interpretation therapy to him.

In order to describe the most important issues that were present towards the end of the play-therapy and thus, the starting point for his art-interpreting therapy, I will give an account of his 19th and 20th session of play-therapy:

In the right half of the sand-box he has built a mighty castle which he identifies with. Along the side of the castle, to the left, is a deep moat, in which lies a crocodile. Above the moat is a big cannon which is built into the castle wall. The cannon is pointing at the Indians who are firing at the castle from the left. One corner of the castle has a shape that probably symbolizes a breast. Here he has placed "a milk-maid." And "a stupid fox is sneaking around the milk-maid." (Previously he has used a fox to symbolize his sister.) Below this "mommy-part" of the castle is the entrance to a cave, which is guarded by a soldier. The boy himself is on his tractor at the top of the mother-part of the castle. This is as far as we get this session,[1] but we continue next time with the reconstruction of the sand-box situation. I explain it to him:

"The castle is you, a part of you, and you have made yourself big and grown up by building a big daddy-cannon into the wall of the castle.

You use it to defend your castle, and yourself ... In the moat lies a crocodile ready to bite, right underneath the cannon — I think you are afraid it will bite you as a punishment for stealing the daddy-cannon. But there is more here — next to the milk-maid, which I think is really Mommy, your sister, of whom you are very jealous, is sneaking around. You yourself are looking after Mommy, and a soldier is guarding the entrance."

He ponders on this for a while, picks up a motor-cross car, and skims the moat where the crocodile is, "drives" into the cave in the Mommy-part of the castle, and says that "it is a garage." The sequence concludes with the motor-cross car attacking the crocodile, "pushing it down on the asphalt with a flame which it sends forth from its rear." Finally the cannon's foundation is reinforced ...

This game is an expression of his mother fixation, sibling

rivalry and castration anxiety. His counter-attack on the castrating agent is of an anal-sadistic nature.

He is in a positive transference situation, and he wants to prolong the therapy sessions and come more often.

In the first art interpreting therapy session, he spontaneously paints in poster colors "a blue tractor on a black road" (Picture no. 1). The tractor appears at the bottom of the sheet, a little to the left. To the right is "a tall, brown mountain." A yellow sun is shining down on the mountain from a blue sky, the tractor's engine is yellow. It is snowing — white brush-strokes fill the sky.

My impression is that this is a rather conventional picture, and I say:

"The pictures are not the most important thing, but the thoughts that strike you when you look at them. What comes to your mind when you look at the tractor, the mountain ... the snow ... can you paint what you are thinking?"

He paints another picture, (no. 2), and starts with an undulating, brown line that runs diagonally from the upper left-hand corner down towards the bottom right-hand corner. It turns into "a mountain," as he fills in the lower area with brown paint. At the top of the mountainside a yellow ball starts rolling downwards. It turns into a larger blue ball, then a green, a red, a white and a brown ball.

"It's the same ball that's rolling, it changes color as it rolls along. And it's raining," he says and paints blue "raindrops' in the air.

"But there's a sun there, too," (in the upper right-hand corner).

I sense a contradiction where the sun and the rain is concerned, and a dramatic quality about the balls that are rolling down the mountain side, and I note:

"It looks like these balls are up to something, what's happening here?"

He follows this up with another picture, no. 3. With a broad brush he draws the outline of "a castle" in black paint. Down below, in the middle of the sheet, appears the entrance, arched, dark brown. A black cannon is looking out from the left-hand side of the castle wall.

"There's lightning in the sky over the castle," he says, as he paints a zig-zag of lightning in yellow. The sun is there, too, above the left-hand tower, shining from a dark blue sky.

I get the impression that this picture is portraying something gloomy and frightening, and ask what it feels like to be him — (the castle, in his earlier sandbox play, represented a part of himself.)

As a response I get the fourth picture this session (Picture no. 4). It represents himself (to the left), and his father inside the castle. "Over Dad's head is a gold lamp," to the right is the arched entrance. Rocket and his father "are sitting at a table drinking."

"What are you drinking?" I ask, having caught his tendency to make things concrete. I get exactly the answer I deserve:

"Dad's drinking beer, and I'm drinking juice."[2]

He starts the next session by painting a series of speed-boats which later proved to be an essential theme in his picture production. In the center "a speed boat that was s'posed to be white." The number 100 refers to the motor's horsepower, the motor is black and oversize (Picture no. 5). He has painted the boat riding on top of the waves in an attempt to create an illusion of speed. He has not been entirely successful, however. The traditional sky gets a deeper shade of blue than usual. Finally the yellow sun appears in the upper left-hand corner.

I ask what comes to his mind:

"A powerful engine, a speed boat? — How is this going to end?"

"Okay, unless . . ."

"Unless what?"

"Unless Dad or I fall in the water and the boat just keeps going, and I don't know what to do — maybe I throw out a lifejacket and he floats over to where the boat is, and I pull him up."

"Sounds like it was Dad who fell in the water?"

"U-hum."

"Maybe you just keep on going?"

He responds with picture no. 6: "Mom and my sister are in the cabin of a jet plane. Dad's the pilot."

It is raining, and the plane is flying towards a rainbow. Rocket grips the brush in a clumsy, uncertain way and holds his breath — he needs to go to the bathroom.

I ask him afterwards if anything came to his mind.
"Nuffin'."
"Is that so! Can you please paint that?"
Whereupon arrives "the volcano!" (Picture no. 7). First a tall, brown mountain that opens at the top to form a volcano. "Red and yellow lava is gushing out." I intensify this:
"Red-hot lava?"
Whereupon the mountain is painted almost all black.
"Black inside?"[3]
"No, on the outside."
"I don't think the last two pictures were so nice either, since we now have a real volcanic eruption! I think you are that red-hot volcano gushing lava!"

Two weeks later (he has been prevented from coming for practical reasons,) he starts with black. It grows into "a big boat, a ferry," (Picture no. 8). I ask what it feels like to be inside.
"Good."
"And who is in charge of making the boat go?"
He doesn't answer, but colors the boat red, as he is saying:
"Nice color, both black and red!"
"U-hum. Are you on your own?"
"With Mom."
"And Dad?"
"He can stay home! It's night-time and we are going to Denmark."
I say:
"Alone on the sea with Mom, and it's night-time ...", whereupon I offer him another sheet of paper.
"Don't try to paint something nice, paint what comes to your mind."
The result is "a white speed-boat" (Picture no. 9) with a large, black outboard motor; the black area is extended to form a cabin.
"The weather is good, and it's day-time."
"For whom?"
"Me and Dad."
"With Mom at night, with Dad in the day-time?"
"Have to go to the bathroom ..."
"Perhaps you can paint what you were thinking, even if it happened a long time ago?"

"U-hum."[4]

It turns into another volcano (Picture no. 10).

"This is your volcano again?"

"Maybe. It just turned out that way."

"It was you who painted it!"

"I got off the boat, and then I saw a volcano with red-hot rocks that came rolling down. Dad was there too."

"Was it dangerous?"

"Yes, red-hot rocks were rolling down on us and we died."

"Both of you?"

"U-hum."

"And then what?"

"Mom and (sister) didn't know what happened to us. They looked, but they couldn't find us. Then they didn't bother to look any more."

"Was it that dangerous?"

"Yeah, we both died!"

Then, a little disconnected:

"He (father) is going full speed to Denmark, takes me with him to go fishing, we go back, then we leave the boat, and then the part about the volcano — then we died." Presently he adds, cautiously:

"(Sister) was alone in the speed-boat."

"Alone?"

"U-hum, but she didn't drown, she did *not* fall in the water!"

"When your sister was born, you were three years old. Can you remember this?"

"I remember I got a whole box of chocolates from Mom."

"Your Mom's very kind! But you were angry anyway?"

"U-hum." (Reserved.)

Because of Easter, I do not see Rocket until three weeks later. I remind him of the birth of his sister, the chocolates his mother gave him, and the fact that his sister did *not* drown (?) — He draws a boat with black outlines this time, it is heading towards the right (Picture no. 11). At the bow is a black antenna. I ask if the number 100 is written backwards.[5]

"It's supposed to be like that 'cause it's going in that direction!"

"What are you thinking about?"

"That my sister and I were going somewhere in this boat."

I remind him that his sister did not drown and say:

"Maybe a painting can show how we think about things that we aren't allowed to think about?"[6]

He picks up another sheet and paints a big jet plane outlined in black (Picture no. 12). It is flying towards the left.

"That's really a powerful one!"

"My sister and I are flying to Denmark, we are going to the 'Tivoli.'" (Fair)

"Can I see that?" (Offering him another sheet.)

His next picture shows a large, brown mountain with a black, looped tunnel (Picture no. 13).

"We are on a roller coaster that's going through a tunnel in this mountain."

"How is it going?"

"Fine, unless (sister) falls out, I have a flash-light, if I saw her falling, I would pull her up again."

"And what if you didn't?"

"Then I wouldn't know what to do ..." (becomes thoughtful).

"Well?"

"I was thinking about a photo of Dad when he was small, he looked a bit funny."

"Small, like you, when your sister was born?"

In the meantime he is on to another picture (Picture no. 14).

"This is us driving a car, after we are grown up."

"We?"

"Me and my sister."

"Who is steering the car?"

"Me."

"I think you have wanted to be big like Daddy for a long time, having your own car! May be when you were small, when your sister was born, you wanted to be big like Daddy and decide over Mommy? But then there would be *two* Daddies?"

The next time I remind him of "being Daddy in relation to Mommy."

"What happened to Daddy?"

"Dad and Mom died."

He paints *Dad is dead*, (Picture no. 15). It begins like this: "Here is the sky", whereupon he paints the upper half in a deep, cobalt blue. The lower part is brown. Buried in this brown "soil" is daddy, in black.

"It's fine if you can paint what comes to your mind!"

He picks up another sheet, and paints almost the same theme, *Mom being dead* (Picture no. 16). He is silent while he paints, with slapping strokes of the brush, a blue sky, a brown earth — "a little less soil".

"What is it going to be?"

"Earth and flowers."

He paints another picture, no. 17.

"This is going to be Daddy — after he's turned into dirt."

He uses brown paint, again with slapping strokes of the brush. Two red and green flowers grow in the brown earth, they are connected to each other.

"These are supposed to grow from the head. A tree is growing from the feet."

The tree is brown with green leaves. He is silent.

"Can you think aloud? What happened to you?"

The speed boat presents itself again in the next picture. It has more speed now, with the keel safely down in the water (Picture no. 18).

"And I was going in the boat, that's me sitting in there, and my hand on the wheel. These are some waves!"

"Looks like you got away!"

"I'm goin' to Denmark, to the fair."

"Looks like you escaped the volcano. And what about your sister?"

"She is at home."

"What about the volcano, the eruption, and the roller-coaster-accident?"

He paints Picture no. 19: A large, brown house with black outlines.

"'Cause then me and my sister got a place to live."

"Together?"

"U-hum."

A purple window, "inside brown walls."

"How are they doing?"

"Fine."

"Is that really true? It doesn't sound like it's true."

He looks at me surprised.

Next time I remind him of the picture-sequence — the death of his father and mother, and finally:

"Was it your sister you went to live with in that brown house, or was it your mother?"

I provide him with pencils and crayons this time:[7]

"Perhaps it's easier for you to use these?"

He draws a red boat that takes off from an island to the right of the picture. There is a flag-pole with a Danish flag on the island. The sky is blue and the sun is shining (Picture no. 20). He says:

"I'm the captain and that's my sister with her arms hanging down, she is relaxing so she won't get so tired."

"Tired?"

"Yes, we take turns steering the boat, but I do it most of the time."

"Is the weather good?"

"Yeah, but we have an awning aboard the boat, and a railing around it."

"So no one can fall out?"

"U-hum."

Another picture, no. 21, with an awning and a strong railing aft. He explains as he goes along:

"In the beginning the weather was good, but then it got bad."

"Like in this picture?"

"It's beginning to rain. (*Blue, short lines.*) It's pouring!"

He continues to draw, but hides the drawing from me.

"Well, then?"

"My sister's at the wheel, and then I raise my arm — like this!" (Lifts his right arm as if to hit something.)

"How did it go?"

"Not too good!"

"Can you draw that?"

He wants another sheet. In his next drawing (no. 22,) the boat has landed, his sister has climbed ashore "with a bad cut on her knee — she's crying." He climbs ashore himself and walks up toward her.

"My sister had to go to the doctor and get a bandage."

He draws some light clouds.

"I think you are making this a little better than it really was?"

"My sister had to go to the hospital ... she used to be able to draw better than me, she once drew a boat that was reflected in the water with many windows ..."

"She was pretty good, then?"

"U-hum." (Resigned.)

We have five sessions left before the summer vacation. I feel that we are at a stand-still:

"Mommy has been missing from your latest pictures. Can you include Mommy in your pictures?"

"Should I draw her dead, with the volcano?"

"Give it a try!"

A new picture: "The brown stuff is dirt," there is a blue sky above it, and green grass is growing in the soil (Picture no. 23).

"Flowers over the spot where Mom and Dad died."

He interrupts himself:

"I need to go to the bathroom."

I ask him to hurry, "because we'll fix this, even if it gets a little scary!"

He goes on to paint two flowers that rise from the ground.

"One is big, the other little?"

"It's like me and my sister." [8]

"How did they get in their Mommy's belly? Can you show me?"

Another picture, no. 24. It is the same brown volcano, but the content is shaped like a red, thick core, which does not penetrate the top. He comments as he goes along:

"At first the volcano erupts, with red-hot rocks coming out of it, then lava pours over Mom and Dad, then them dies, and their ashes turn into dirt, and two flowers grow up from the dirt."

"Can you paint a picture with just Daddy in it?"

On another sheet: *When I was Daddy* (Picture no. 25). In an ingenious way he demonstrates how he is changed into Daddy. First he paints himself, (to the right), then a couple of symbols for movement, (Z-signs, the symbols are barely visible between the two figures.) Then comes Daddy, "with a big nose" (to the left.) He explains that he "sort of gets up and changes into Daddy."

"Can you paint more about what it is like being Daddy?"

"Can I just draw Daddy?"

"That's too easy! You as Daddy."

"Draw me and Daddy?"

"Why don't you ask yourself!"

It turns into a large, brown car that takes up almost all of the lower half of the sheet (Picture no. 26). He himself, painted as a large, black head, is sitting at the wheel "with a nose as big as Daddy's, a black antenna and riding on a bumpy road."[9]

I demonstrate the rocking movements of a car on a bumpy road. He smiles.

"I guess you have a big penis too, then?"

He paints yellow flames gushing out of "a fire-pipe under the car." Above it are "speed-stripes", also in yellow.

"I see that you have wished you were Daddy, Mommy's sweetheart. You wished you could decide over Mommy's body, with only you there, and not your sister. Be the boss of everything in the whole world!"

Joyfully he runs out to the waiting room, while showing how far he can slide on his socks.

The next time he arrives, there is a new quickness about him. He is able to organize the paint and brushes better. Spontaneously he asks to see the drawings from last time.

Then he proceeds to paint a "summer house" (Picture no. 27). He tells me that his family went to their summer house for the Whitsun holidays. (Wishful thinking, according to his father, who came to pick the boy up after the session.) "The summer house is made of nice, broad panelling," it has a porch and a door, and the door has a bright yellow window with a shining star above it in the same color." The roof has red, curved tiles.

"I think you're painting a summer house for sweet-hearts."[10]

He nods and paints a blue sky and a yellow sun, whereupon he starts painting on another sheet, the same summer house, now close to the water (Picture no. 28). The speed-boat is here, lying quietly in front of the summer house with an outboard motor and "speed-lines."

"I think you would like to stay here for ever."

Quickly he sketches: a black boat, "out in the tall waves — and there is a cloud in front of the sun." (Picture no. 29). I say:

"The sea is mother whom you command with the black boat.

The sun, which is now growing dark with anger, is your father."[11]

Next time he wishes to see his previous pictures again, and I ask for the continuation, "the way only you can paint it." He holds his breath and starts painting:

"Me and the boat ... with pants (blue) ... and a sweater (red) ..."

The face is drawn in black paint, the hair is red, in his hand he is holding a brown fishing rod with the line hanging out (Picture no. 30).

"I think you have made yourself stronger with a long penis!"

He needs to go to the bathroom. Presently I say:

"The sea is mother and the sun, Daddy, is not here. That means you are out fishing in the Mommy-sea. You are Mommy's sweetheart, with a long penis, like Daddy's."

Rocket nods, while at the same time squirting blue paint from the bottle onto the picture from the right:[12]

"The sea is whirled up by the motor in the back."

The next picture depicts *A new boat with a first mate* (Picture no. 31). The "speed-stripes" are now "real flames". It is raining on one side (to the right), on the other side is "nice, warm sunlight," painted with red and yellow stripes. The ocean is heaving with tall waves.

"There is more sun here than rain," he says.

"Wishful thinking?"

"U-hum."

"The sea is Mommy, the sun is Daddy, and you are a powerful boat. It's both sunny and rainy, and you are riding on tall waves ...?"

He draws the same theme in a new edition: a red, powerful racing car (Picture no. 32), with "speed lines" and the number 75, races in from the right with Rocket at the wheel.

"I own this car! There's no rain here!"

"Only sunshine and happiness — quite a wish!" He adds more yellow sunbeams.

We have two sessions left. I let him look at, and comment on, two pictures which I have selected:

First *Daddy disguised as a rocket* — an easel painting in watercolor from the first observation session — I haven't given an account of it here. It is a phallus in disguise. He doesn't recognise the picture,[13] but comes to think of something that he wants to paint: It is another phallus, "a pillar," something he "has seen at the place where Daddy works." (Picture no. 33).

"Both Daddy disguised as a rocket and this pillar mean, in the language of dreams, the grown-up daddy-penis that you have been wishing for."

Afterwards I show him the "speed-boat that is out in the sun and rain." He obviously recognizes it, and draws in pencil and crayons a similar picture. The sun and the rain are connected by a rainbow that stretches out across almost the whole of the sheet.[14]

I interpret this as an expression of increased integration, of a softening of the conflict between the aggressive castration-wish and the fear of punishment, and I say:

"I think you are reconciled with Daddy — and especially with Mommy. You are going to let Daddy be Daddy and Mommy be Mommy! You are good enough just the way you are!"

We have arrived at our last session. I bring out the rainbow picture:

"Is there something else that you want to paint?"

He draws with pencil and crayon (Picture no. 35) the same boat with zig-zags on the side, but now "the motor is inside the boat." He is "alone, the sea is calm —"

"How very nice!"

Then follows on another sheet of paper: *An island with a palm tree and blue sea* (Picture no. 36). The boat is landing at the island, he is fastening it to "a huge rock." "Nobody lives there — only me." He draws "a trembling figure": it "was so hot — and he got an electric shock that came from far away, his hair is standing on end, his body is shaking."

"And then what?"

He draws the boat heading homewards, to pick up his sister (Picture no. 37).

"We are going to the palm-island together, on vacation!"

In his last picture, (no. 38) the boat is returning to the island "me and Mommy alone on our way to the palm-island, without my sister." (Wistful.)

The parents were pleased with his conduct at home at this point, the attacks on his mother had ceased. They wanted me to recommend an increase in the special tutoring programme in school.

BEYOND WORDS

Notes to Narrative

1. The situation illustrates how troublesome and time-consuming it is for him to construct such an intricate situation. It leaves no time to work through the issues. If one later wishes to return to a particular sequence, one has nothing visual to refer to, and one must meticulously reconstruct the whole scene.
2. The picture is produced in a state of introspection. It is a projection of pre-conscious material, and the execution reflects this; it is sketchy, with a simple color scheme — reddish brown and yellow, and multi-determined in its expressive content.
3. At this point I have a distinct notion that the black paint represents a growing fear of retaliation, and I want him to "taste" this feeling, not just project the anxiety and treat it like an outside matter.
4. Here I helped him by offering distance through the phrase "a long time ago," hoping that this would improve his introspective ability.
5. He is reading the number as if seen through a mirror, a part of his dyslexia.
6. The dream wish behind his notion that his sister didn't die, does not contain the negative "didn't". See S. Freud: *The Interpretation of dreams*, part II, p. 43: "The manner in which the dream deals with the categories 'contradiction' and 'contrast' is extraordinary. The two are simply ignored. 'No' as a concept seems to be non-existent in the world of dreams."
7. I introduce pencils and crayons to tone down his involvement somewhat, hoping thus to obtain more pre-conscious material.
8. I associate here the fact that both he and his sister have been carried and given birth to by his mother, as an outcome of the following line of thought: mother dies, out of the soil that mother has become, two flowers grow. — After I have emphasized that one of the flowers is bigger than the other, he associates the fact that the flowers represent himself and his sister. Also implied in his statement is, I believe, the following: "I am assaulting mother's life-giving ability and

the fact that she has carried and given birth to another child in addition to me." Thus I am coaxing him back to the original sibling conflict.
9. The nose here symbolizes a penis, and the theme is a sexual act.
10. The "hut" (summer house), as it was painted and described when he recounted his imagined experiences of the Whitsun holidays, unquestionably represented his mother.
11. The ocean, "la mer," is an archaic mother-symbol. The sun has often symbolized father, at least in patriarchal cultures. I consider the speed-boat to be a penis-symbol. (Freud, Drommetydning (*The Interpretation of Dreams*,) part II, p. 75: "All complicated machinery and appliances that appear in dreams most probably represent genitals — usually male, and in its description of these the dream symbolism is as untiring as the art of making jokes."
12. His destructive self assertion has repeatedly manifested itself through anal expressions. He kills the castrating crocodile with flames from the car's rear, he frequently abuses his mother with anal obscenities. The brown volcano is, as far as color and functioning is concerned, an anal-sadistic symbol.
13. The failure to recognize an earlier picture often means that the conflict has been solved, or at least mitigated, thus rendering the picture obsolete or insignificant.
14. A rainbow, when used in poetry, art and in art therapy, is often regarded as a symbol of family conflicts or as a bridge between contradictory feelings.

DISCUSSION

DIAGNOSTIC

Rocket (8½ years old) has a serious learning disability, complicated by dyslectic problems and delayed psycho-motor development. He behaves in an uncontrolled and destructive manner, especially at home in relation to his mother. His gross motor functioning is clumsy, his fine motor functioning is also impaired and his reading-writing deficiencies call for a more thorough investigation by a special education teacher.

Play observation reveals an ambivalent mother-fixation, intense sibling rivalry, and a relatively overt castration anxiety. His aggression has an anal-sadistic quality.

He is trusting and it is easy to establish a situation of positive interaction with him, but his development is held back because his natural drive to explore is inhibited. His general intellectual functioning is good and he receives adequate stimulation at home. His sister, who is three years younger, is lively and mature for her age.

After 24 sessions of play therapy he has displayed his infantile conflicts through sand-box play without obtaining any significant relief from this activity. The reasons are his concretizing tendency and his difficulties in expressing himself through abstract and complex language.

THERAPEUTIC GOAL

To alleviate his neurotically based learning disability, it is necessary to install in him a more "digestible" image of an internalized mother, projected and reintrojected through a transference situation.

The sibling rivalry is closely tied to his relationship to his mother and therefore the treatment of both these issues will overlap.

His father-rivalry is rather overt, and will therefore probably prove to be the most accessible issue therapeutically. More profoundly, this feeling of rivalry is liable to respond favorably to a softening of the destructive conflict with his mother.

In Freudian terms, a change in the inner balance between id, ego and super-ego, increased tolerance to their individual goals, and thus a more harmonious interaction between them, would be the ultimate goal of this therapy. But a thorough analytic process of such a nature is not feasible here for practical reasons.

THERAPEUTIC METHOD

He needed an artistic medium suitable for the projection of multi-determined, revived images. This medium must be

interesting for him to work with; it should not be anxiety-provoking and it should further this special form of transference — the projection of infantile material in a transference relationship (a sub-species of the transference process proper.[1])
I arrived at this conclusion after assuming that his intellectually disabling conflicts were subject to primary repression and that the dream wishes were of a preverbal nature which he would be unable to describe verbally.

For the above mentioned reasons, and also to increase the depth of experience and to discourage his inclination to view issues in concrete terms only, art interpreting therapy was introduced after 24 sessions of play therapy.

Initially his artistic endeavours were marked by his tendency to think in concrete terms, and by his sluggish disposition and poorly developed imagination.

His positive relationship to me is further enhanced during this stage. More than a transference person, he now counts on me as a person to identify with. He produces several significant pictorial sequences, i.e. the presentation of the injuring of his sister; the death and burial of his mother and father; his wish to be daddy and possess his virile powers, ("when I was Daddy,") along with his wish to be the destructive master of his mother's body.

The most valuable result of the therapy is the beneficial effect obtained from externalizing the latent dream wishes in a pictorially projected form. The pictures are handed to the therapist, an act which serves to bring about the process of transference. He creates the projections himself, and as time goes by, he perceives these to be an expression of his own thoughts and feelings. The therapist is functioning as an auxilliary ego. This is a source of strength to him, for instance when he is externalizing his wish to be the destructive master of Mommy's body — a wish which one supposes must have been subjected to primary repression.

His excessive, destructive aggression towards his mother ceases as a result of the therapy. In Freudian terms, this is an effect of his having used me as a vehicle for free-floating libido, disconnected from the mother-object.[2]

In all probability he had earlier sought to diminish his overwhelming sense of guilt by invoking as much scolding, correction and punishment as possible from his mother. The effect of the therapy is that the pressure from his super-ego is relieved, the relationship between his super ego and ego has been harmonized, and his relationship to his mother has again become libidinized. In addition, his ego has been strengthened by his creative activities.

Throughout the therapy he has indirectly been confronted with the fact that his infantile reaction pattern is no longer adequate. His parents have supported him through the whole of the therapy, emphatically and patiently, never shying away from great physical efforts to enable him to go through with the therapy. They have picked him up after each session, and the experience of the contrast between the infantile quality of the therapy-sessions and the reality out in the waiting room and in every-day life has contributed to his previously uncontrolled id-impulses being increasingly more controlled by his ego.

Notes to Discussion

1. Anna Freud: *Normality and Pathology in Childhood.* Assessment of Development. (1966), pp. 41 – 43:
   "Not all the relations established or transferred by a child in analysis are object relations in the sense that the analyst becomes cathected with libido or aggression. Many are due to externalizations, i.e., to processes in which the person of the analyst is used to represent one or the other part of the patient's personality structure. So far as the analyst "seduces" the child by tolerating freedom of thought, fantasy, and action (the latter within limits), he becomes the representative of the patient's id, . . . So far as he verbalizes and helps in the fight against anxiety, he becomes an auxiliary ego to whom the child clings for protection. Due to his being an adult, the analyst is seen and treated by the child also as an external superego, i.e. paradoxically as a moral judge of the very derivatives which have been liberated by his efforts. The child thus re-stages his internal (intersystemic) conflicts as external battles with the analyst, a process which provides useful material. To interpret such externalizations in terms of object relationship within the transference would

be a mistake, even though originally all conflicts within the structure have their source in earliest relationships. At the time of therapy, however, their importance lies in the fact that they reveal what happened in a child's inner world, in the relations between his inner agencies, as contrasted with the emotional relationships to objects in the external world ... Understood in this manner, externalization is a subspecies of transference. Treated as such in interpretation and kept separate from transference proper, it is a valuable source of insight into the psychic structure."

2. Anna Freud: *Normality and Pathology in Childhood*, p. 233: "Destructive tendencies which have become excessive due to defusion of libido and aggression are lessened and bound again, if libidinal attachments are promoted. The libidinal and aggressive processes themselves answer to the offer of an object for cathexis. Ego attitudes are changed where opportunities for identification are opened up, or superego pressure relieved by opportunity for suitable externalization."

3   Black Rhomb

NARRATIVE

Black Rhomb was 20 years old when I proposed art interpreting therapy.

Six months earlier I had had her hospitalized in a psychiatric ward because of an acute paranoid psychosis. After a two months' stay the hospital wanted me to take over the treatment. Her psychosis was well controlled, she had received antipsychotic drug treatment as well as regular supportive counselling.

I had meetings with her parents where we discussed her situation and I agreed to start weekly therapy sessions with their daughter. I reduced her medication to a minimum.

After a few therapy sessions, Black Rhomb was still in a severely depressed state. She stayed at home, isolated and apathetic. She felt sad and dejected and did not think that our therapy sessions had improved her situation.

Her mother despaired over her daughter's situation — she just stayed at home, resigned, completely lacking initiative.

Her father thought that the situation was getting worse — "she is obviously suffering, she is totally unsocial, can't bring herself to go out and see people, can't get started in the job I have found for her."

Black Rhomb was the older of two children, her brother was 4 years younger. Her mother thought that "he always had been more affectionate" — he was a happy and healthy senior high student.

After 12 supportive sessions, I found the time ripe to end her drug treatment and begin art interpreting therapy — we agreed on 1 to 2 sessions a week until the summer — about 10 sessions and a summing up with the possibility of continuing when summer was over.

When she arrives for her first session, she insists that she can neither paint nor draw. Previously she has drawn some pictures for me using colored pencils and I show her these drawings. The sketches are the results of her efforts to draw naturalistic human figures. The figures are simple stereotypes. It is clear to both of us that the naturalistic form of drawing is difficult for her. We agree to try to find a more suitable non-figurative mode with emphasis on colors and their internal relationships.

I suggest fingerpainting. Her first picture, *The Experiment* (Picture No. 1), is the result of testing out the possibilities of fingerpainting. While she is trying out various techniques, I encourage her to be especially aware of what the specific colors mean to her, resulting in the following color scheme: **red and black** represent the strongest emotions: **yellow** stands for longing; **brown** represents disgusting things: **blue and green** stand for beauty and clarity.

Next I encourage her to "think Mommy," (Picture no. 2). She starts out with a deep, blue color. This gets painted over with a black square standing on edge, the shape of a rhomb. In the middle a bright yellow area. The original blue paint shines through a slot along the bottom of the rhomb.

"This is my mother," she says.

To the right she paints three tiny red fuzz-balls:

"This is us trying to get in touch with mother."

The whole scene is framed by a red arch, resembling the outline of a cave. The area surrounding the 'cave' is green.

"It looks like it is difficult to get in touch with mother. (*I point to the black rhomb*) But something is shining inside it! (*I point to the yellow area in the center*) You said yellow stands for longing. (*Pointing to the three red fuzz-balls:*[1]) It looks like the others had trouble reaching her too!"

She is alert but silent.

"I think you always longed for mother!"

I ask her to paint a picture of the whole family together.[2] The next picture, Picture no. 3, consists of colored geometric shapes. Father is brown, rectangular, and standing on edge. Mother is a black square. She herself is the larger red circle. She and mother are placed in the center of the picture, father is situated close to mother in the upper left-hand corner. Underneath mother and father is the brother, represented by a smaller circle.

This is a premeditated composition. I go through the choice of colors and placement with her, while at the same time emphasizing the various shapes:

"Both parents are angular, the children are round. If you

look at the placement and choice of colors simultaneously, it is like a song in two voices, with you and mother in the center. The two of you are the most intense colors, red and black."

She makes no comment, and I leave it at that.

We have decided on 2 sessions weekly in the beginning, "to get off to a good start." She drops by two days after the initial session to cancel her next appointment, the reason being that she has been sick all night and that she is still "nauseous and in poor shape." It seems to be a physical condition, and I make an appointment to see her the following day. She seems more motivated than before.

When she arrives for her next appointment, she takes her time with her first picture (Picture no. 4). She starts out with the circle, and her face has a dreamy, evanescent expression. I ask what is on her mind.

"The argument with mother." (She points to the circle.)

"How?"

"Right out of the blue, she slapped my face. But worst of all were the apologies afterwards!"

She is busy painting the green area that is curling up close to the violet patch in the bottom right-hand corner.

"This is out in the world — I wish I was far away!"

Both the doctor at the hospital and myself felt that her sudden attempt to break away from her mother was very important — the event that had triggered her psychotic breakdown. Therefore I say:

"I think you should find a way out of the circle first."

I point to the original part of the picture, the circle with the yellow center, to the decreasingly intense red area surrounding it, and to the black, hard outer shell. I describe it to her thus, and she says,

"Nice warm core? — No, only a black, hard shell!"

Aside from this picture, the session is not very productive. Instead I am confronted with a long string of complaints — everything is hopeless, just staying at home, not being able to get out! I point to my watch:

"Your wailing is taking up all the time that was supposed to be spent painting!"

Next week I show her her last picture.

"Perhaps you were a little angry with this hard, black shell?"

She responds with *The vigorous, blue wheel*, a design with a blue, round center that radiates blue beams which are cut short by a blue outer circle (Picture no. 5).

"Well?"

"It's radiating, but the rays are stopped by a wall, Mom and Dad!"

Her eyes come alive while she is talking. I commend her on the positive element that seems to be present in the center of this "wheel of protest."

"Please paint this positive element!"

She paints two red figures, the upper parts of the bodies, only, (Picture no. 6). The bodies are close together, arms around each other, — "the air is bright around them, they are free, not confined!" She adds:

"It's *not* me!"

"Your eyes certainly were alive a moment ago!"

I remind her of our agreement that she should associate freely while I, on my part, will maintain complete discretion.

"Perhaps this picture has something of you in it after all?"

She looks at me and smiles, a little surprised.

"I don't think these red figures have a sex-life, the lower part of their bodies is missing."[3]

She seems to be in a good mood, almost elated, when she arrives for her next appointment.

"Are you on a pink cloud today?"

"I'm both happy and realistic."

I remind her of her picture from last time and comment on the good contact she conveys.

"I think you put it very precisely, 'both happy and realistic.' But perhaps there is something you still wish for?"

She responds by painting *The pink cloud*, a large, pink cloud on a blue sky with green grass underneath (Picture no. 7).

"Yes, that's it, but can you try to clarify it, put more of you in it?"

The next picture she calls *The bar against the outside world* (Picture no. 8). The sheet is divided in half by a vertical red line. To the left she paints first *The Splitting-up*.

"Red is separated from Blue, like shell from core, — and this is separated from the red on the outside" (she points).

On the other side of the red line are "lots of living people."

I commend her on her precise manner of expressing the psychotic split feeling she has experienced.

"And you said you couldn't paint! I think you have done an excellent job of presenting your experiences!"

The next time she comes, I encourage her to present her relationship to father. She paints father like a round, brown patch in the upper right-hand corner (Picture no. 9). On top of it "something black and obstructing." She paints herself in the lower left-hand corner, "something red with the blind pulled down." (The black top-layer.)

"Did you have anything specific in mind?"

"It could have been 'Equality in love,' she says with a sigh.

"Please paint that."

Picture No. 10 is a non-figurative repetition of Picture no. 6, with the two red figures close together.

"Perhaps you could paint 'being small'?"[4]

A round yellow field is "safely embraced" by a green area (Picture no. 11).

"Yellow stands for small and active."

A sharp, black line penetrates the green area. To the right of the black line is "father — blue, hard and wise."

"Was it just safe?"

She answers with Picture no. 12, "When father shut himself off." She paints herself "black with lots of prickles."

"I slam the door on him and walk to my brother's room."

The art-work is now becoming more and more like a cartoon-strip, and her next picture is: *Myself beating my fists at Daddy,* in red and black, like a double zig-zag of lightning! (Picture no. 13).

"Is it both angry and destructive?"

"No, it is 'love-red' and 'angry-black.'"

"Love-hate?"

"U-humm."

"You have rendered this subject very well! Do you feel the difference between painting a spontaneous picture and painting something the way you think it is supposed to look?"

"Sometimes it's a little of each, but this time the composition just 'happened'."

Next time I pick up on her relationship to father and encourage her to paint a new expression of this theme. The picture (no. 14) develops into a continuation of Picture no. 9, where she had placed her father and herself diagonally across from each other. This time there is no overpainting, father is a brown blotch in the upper right-hand corner, Black Rhomb herself in blue in the lower left-hand corner. A vigorous, violet line connects the two blotches. She says:

"We are growing more apart all the time."

"Strange then, that you have joined the two of you here (*I point to the violet line*) — what do you think of that?"

She responds by painting another picture, (no. 15). First there is " a red egg and a yellow area. The yellow is squeezed out by the red egg."

"And the green field?"

"That's the world around us."

"Once before you painted the positive aspect of a mother as yellow — the kindness that you longed for — but here you fight it off! Perhaps you wish that you yourself were mother? Please go on painting."

Her last picture on this occasion (no. 16): a fat, black worm arching across the center of the page. Vigorous blue beams radiating from a blue center at the bottom of the sheet.

"The blue beams are me, and you are the black worm pressing down on me, but the blue beams are holding up against it without collapsing. They are forcing their way upwards, trying to shed the black, oppressing element. Is it possible to defeat the black worm — or will the whole thing break down and turn into earth and dust," she wonders.

She is completely carried away by the description. My impression is that this dream is a battle against an earlier sexual transgression, and I support her in her fierce resistance.

She calls me before her next appointment to say "I can't come, the vacation is right around the corner and I have got a summer job."

"You have told me some things that you would rather forget about, perhaps — I think you ought to come, it's the last time before the vacation starts."

But she insists that she has to show up at work, and we agree to continue in the fall.

This part of the therapy, from January until June, has consisted of 20 sessions, the last 8 sessions with art interpreting therapy. The last part of the therapy, lasting from the middle of August till the middle of October, consists of 9 art interpreting therapy sessions. We continued the therapy after being urged to do so by Black Rhomb's father.

Her father contacted me early in the fall to ensure the continuation of his daughter's therapy. He related some detailed information about Black Rhomb's early development: She was very active as an infant, crawling from the time she was six months old, walking when she was one. She disturbed her parents' sleep during the first couple of years of her life by climbing into their bed at night. She was breastfed with a supplement of baby formula till she was 4 months old, when she was abruptly weaned. At three years of age she went through a spell of not wanting to eat. This lasted about a week. Her mother was pregnant with Black Rhomb's brother when this happened.

Black Rhomb shows up as planned. I suggest 2 sessions a week if possible — she has a permanent job, but is going to try to arrange this anyway.

She has a little trouble getting started with her first picture and tries a blue cloud in the upper left-hand corner, (Picture no. 17), whereupon she arrives at the conclusion that "there are really only two possibilities." This she demonstrates by painting a scale of colors at the top of the sheet, black, blue, white, red and yellow, with an all black splotch at the bottom.

"It looks like you are trying to express 'either — or!' Life is rarely like that."

"But this is what it feels like."

"As in the picture, up in the clouds, happy and colorful, or down in the pits, black and somber? — If anything comes to your mind, please paint it."

Another picture, she calls it *Oppression* (Picture no. 18). First "a bird's wing, closing down over something but failing to suffocate it completely."

"'Something is being suffocated?' That sounds rather vague!"

"Yes, I just can't seem to finish it —"

"Unfinished Composition?"

She accepts the challenge and asks for another sheet of paper.

The theme is carried further in her new picture, Picture no. 19.

"It's not coming so close this time," is my comment.

"No, the last time mother had joined father (*the suffocating wing,*) this time it's father only. He is a little more practical, keeps at a distance."

"First this small creature, then a practical father somewhere out in the periphery."

"This is really hard to draw — but it's supposed to be a bird. (*She dresses up the wing a little.*) The bird is farther away from me here, there is more air between us," she adds.

"Mother leaves you more with a feeling of being choked, perhaps? You often talk about her 'grinding way of caring'."

She sighs, but seems relieved at the same time.

"And then what?"

"I wish I could run away from it all!"

"Paint it!"

And she paints "a happy red 'broad', with her close friends down there (*red blotch.*)"

"And the blue stuff over in that corner is mother and father." (Picture no. 20).

This is a clearly premeditated composition, but still bubbling with life and a catching rhythm and motion. The effect that this picture has on her causes her to finish her session with, for the first time, a "Thank you — see you later!"

When she arrives the next time, I encourage her to paint "that which is holding you back, the most personal, the most 'Black Rhomb'ish' of everything you have in you!"

She paints a human figure, "this is myself," above it some dots, "those are people, and then there is a small black area inside me." (Picture no. 21).

"How do you really get on with other people?"

"I withdraw from them."

"Yes, I think you are right. I think you reject in order to avoid being rejected. — Can you please paint the opposite?"

"Not withdrawing?"

"Yes."

Picture no. 22: "A lot of people doing fun things, — or, not necessarily a lot of people." She draws two small blue fingures between two larger ones.

"It looks like a mother and a father and two children? What do you think will happen now?"

Picture no. 23: another cartoon, and she explains:

"If I become more outgoing, and more open to other people, my feelings might get hurt, somebody might let me down and I might lose my self-confidence."

The pink rhomb, which has a head, is filled in which many colors, a whole scale of colors. To the right is the upper part of a body, black and in the shape of a rhomb. It has both a head and a trunk. I ask what is inside the black frame. (The situation had been on the verge of becoming a trite serial because of her habit of putting herself down.)

The non-figurative composition which is presented in her next picture (Picture no. 24) she calls *Flames or oil or something like that is pouring out from openings all over the body.* I point to the fact that both red and black are represented here:

"Which you called 'the colors of love and hate.' In the middle you have painted the color of longing, yellow, but also the color of sadness, violet."

Time is up.

Next time I pick up the thread from the previous session — the colorful jet of flames and oil. She paints a new picture, (no. 25) which she names *Confrontation, negative from the start.* Two black figures in a close fight. An air of combat surrounds the scene, made visible by vivid red strokes.

Black Rhomb has a habit of painting a naturalistic composition when she makes her first picture after arriving for her therapy sessions. I encourage her to find another mode of expression which is not dependant on a naturalistic execution. She paints Picture no. 26, "it is supposed to be from my diary — the black represents home," she starts out from the left:

"A passionate moment, the way I felt it . . . (*the black and the red paint becomes intermeshed,*) . . . and it all ends up in red flames, I burn all my diaries, especially because of the passion, the physical sensation, and especially when it comes to Mommy and Daddy."

"It seems like something needs to be kept from mother and father, we will go through that next time."

Next time she spontaneously proceeds to paint *The Burning of the Diary.* I get the impression that she is moving on several levels: first she paints two vigorous, undulating strokes with her finger, "an eel or something like that." The undulating lines are in black and red, the color of hate and love. (Picture no. 27).

"But there is something else as well," she says, and draws a green and a blue wave on top of the others.

"You said blue was clear and lovely, and perhaps green stands for growth, and now you are adding these to the colors of love and hate."

She proceeds with another sheet of paper, and the next picture is: *A Leap out into the All Red* (Picture no. 28). A figure in the shape of a fish is "fleeing to the left." Following close behind is a large, black, similar figure.

"Now it's turned all black again — Mommy, (*black fish*) is trying to swallow me! But I can be just as black, and then I push her away!"

She paints the opposite situation, (Picture no. 29): A rhomb that eventually turns all black. Mother is represented by a smaller "red fish that's fleeing." I commend her on her simple, precise expression.

"And you are the strong one now. Mother is smaller, on the run. But are you really happy about it?"

I begin the next session with: "The strong, black, angry element is a part of you, but perhaps you are something else as well? Something warm and close, like here and now?"

Referring to the expression on her face and the look in her eyes, I say:

"I don't see anything black, angry or punishing in your eyes."

She starts painting in black and red, (Picture no. 30) and says:

"This is also here-and-now, but it is surrounded by Black — almost."

She has completed the black and the red areas now, leaving a narrow opening at the top! I describe the composition to her:

"Black is almost taking over, but not completely."

I go on to describe the three levels on which I think she finds herself now and make my own drawing: three double waves alternating between black and red; one is the small child level, the second: the level of dawning sexuality. The third level is the here-and-now. (See footnote 3).

"Can you please paint how *you* feel about this?"

She paints another picture (no. 31) and calls it *Myself, the ideal* picture of me. I am one quarter black, the rest of it red — which is what holds me together."

At this point her mother asks advice for herself, and I am informed about two central issues in this family. Her first child died as an infant one year before Black Rhomb was born, thus her next child became a substitute. When she was six months pregnant with Black Rhomb, her own father also died. She had been very attached to him. In addition she was able to confirm that Black Rhomb was breastfed with a supplement of baby formula until she was four months old, when suddenly there was no more breast milk.

I wish now to work through the ambivalent relationship to mother, and start the next session thus:

"What is it that you are always pushing aside, and how do you do it? Please try to show in it a painting!"

She paints a figure outlined in black, (Picture no. 32) — "a head-body", then "something inside too, there must be something there because I have some really hysterical outbursts at times!"

"I think you can make it even clearer."

She makes another attempt, Picture no. 33. This is a larger edition of the same black figure, but "a dragon spouting flames" has now invaded the lower half of the figure.

"I think you have, in your picture, put yourself back into your mother's womb, and that you are about to break loose, be born again, so to speak!"

She responds by painting (Picture no. 34): "A small, round lump that's running away, bustling, cross, and with a lot of spunk! I don't need a mother any more — not one who cares about me in such a way ... it was the way she did it, not that I wanted her to die or anything!"

We have two sessions left, and use them to sum it all up. But first she tells me about her work and her future plans, showing increased insight and realism. Then she paints a prompted picture — an expression of her own development. (Picture no. 35). In the bottom left-hand corner "as a very small child, black, boisterous, a real rascal", then "a school-girl, much nicer," in blue. Then follows a "high-school girl with a freakish style," then "Freaky all the way." But then the fun is over, and she is "black and small, back to where I started."

"Okay, but that little girl was quite rebellious! Next time we'll talk about that rebellious little girl!"

The main theme of her last session: "Adjusting in spite of the conditions", as she puts it, illustrating her point with Picture no. 36. It gradually becomes a softly undulating scale of colors in green, pink, blue, yellow, black and light pink.[5]

"What a beautiful integration of colors!"

Her mother relates during a conversation some months later that her daughter is now doing well in a permanent job.

Notes to Narrative

1. I was told later that the mother had borne 3 children; an older daughter died 3 weeks old, 1 year before the birth of Black Rhomb. This explains "The three tiny, red, fuzzy balls."
2. Because she has recently been through a psychotic stage, I took more of a leading role when it came to choice of themes than I would in the treatment of a neurosis, and was more supportive of all constructive activity.
3. I knew that she had had an *abortus provocatus* shortly before she went into psychosis, and assumed that this had had an influence on her abrupt attempt to separate herself from her mother, the factor which had triggered the paranoid psychosis.
4. To give the pictures a name or a short text has two advantages: the patient may create some distance between herslef and the picture, as in an art exhibition; it also has a mobilizing effect on the preconscious images because it stimulates a person to enter a daydreaming state of mind.
5. A color scheme consisting of these colors in many cases seems to be an expression of increased personal integration. (See Margaret Naumburg: *An Introduction to Art Therapy*.)

DISCUSSION

DIAGNOSTIC

Black Rhomb — a 20 year old girl — is in a seriously depressed state after having recently gone through a paranoid-psychotic phase. The onset of the psychosis was probably triggered by an abrupt attempt at releasing herself from an invasive attachment to her internalized mother, and intensified by a recent *abortus provocatus*.

I assumed that her paranoid psychosis was rooted in her earliest psycho-sexual development, and that she had, during the hospital stay, been helped to move from "the paranoid-schizoid position" (Melanie Klein) to "the depressive position," but had been left here unable to emerge from her depressed state.[1].

THERAPEUTIC GOAL

The goal now must be to let her, preferably through an externalizing process, re-experience some of the hateful feelings that had been veiled by the depressed state. A different, non-invasive, positive therapy situation had to be established to make this possible.

Through such means I could expect to soften the paralyzing tendency to depression and mobilize her capacity to enter a positive relationship to a new object of identification.

The prerequisite for reliving the hopelessness and feeling of loss at a preverbal stage of development must be a form of therapy where non-verbal elements play the main part.

The alternative to such a mode of treatment was in reality a long-term verbal ego-supporting therapy, possibly combined with anti-depressant medication. A psycho-analytical form of treatment was not practically and economically within reach.

A minimum goal must be to get her sufficiently activated for her to be able to continue with her studies or get started in a suitable job.

THERAPEUTIC METHOD

The first 12 sessions consisted of verbal ego-supporting psychotherapy with gradual reduction of her anti-psychotic medication.

The next 15 sessions consisted of art interpreting psychotherapy with finger painting 1 – 2 times a week as needed.

For the art interpreting therapy I will aim at non-figurative expression, with emphasis on the various colors. I will regard colors and their composition to be the most important graphic element besides lines and values, and the element which gives to the picture its hallmark, and thus its experiential value.

This therapy represented a great challenge to the method. Her apathy and lack of self-confidence were main factors — she was "no good, she was not able to express herself, especially not through painting, had never been good at drawing," etc. Her pictures were not very "interesting" therapeutically, the treatment was not dramatic or exciting. What little artistic talent she might possess, was effectively held back by the feeling of uselessness caused by her depression.

In her first explorative picture she works out her palette, what the specific colors and color combinations symbolize for her, emotionally. Her palette closely resembled "The ancient tradition in color symbolism" (Margaret Naumberg, 1973).

In her next picture, a "prompted" picture where I ask her to "think" mother, she is projecting her main inner conflict symbolized by the black unapproachable rhomb and, in contrast, the small, yearning yellow area in the center.

This picture is obviously produced in a premeditated state of mind. Nevertheless, from an expressionistic point of view, it is also well composed. It effectively conveys the attraction to the longed for object, and the binding is well expressed through the embracing red "cave" which surrounds the theme. Characteristically her main inner conflict is presented in an initial picture. One may assume that it is the first time she has been given the opportunity to express this conflict in a symbolic, artistic form which is more descriptive than a lot of complaining words.

Comparing this with Picture no. 24, *Fire and Oil*, where she expresses her need to change the conditions, one may infer that she has experienced a not insignificant support of her ego in the intervening sessions. This picture is more spontaneous, an unambiguous composition of a more pre-conscious nature. The form is loose, her latent artistic talent is emerging. The movement in this pictorial expression indicates a powerful outburst. The content is conveyed to the therapist in a transference situation, and it is reasonable to assume that a significant improvement has taken place.

The first protest against the invasive and binding aspect in the relationship to her mother appears in Picture no. 33 where she has painted a black uterine symbol with "a fire-spitting dragon" inside. The picture arrives as a result of a further development of the motif that was presented in the preceding picture. I interpret it to mean that "she is forcing her way out of her mother's womb, being reborn," and her response arrives directly, in the shape of "a small, round ball flying off somewhere, shrewish and with a lot of spunk." In addition she has a verbal response:

"I don't need a mother any more — at least not when this is her way of showing that she cares. Not that I wish her dead or anything ..."

(The last part, the negation of the death wish, confirms my interpretation and reflects her effort to let it sink back into a repressed state.)

In Freudian terms, her excessive aggression, which among other things was caused by an abrupt weaning at the age of 4 months, had released a surplus of decathected libido, and this decathected libido had responded to the offer of a new object of cathection, the therapist. The excessive aggression is thus subdued, and the attitude of the ego is altered as a response to the offer of a new object of identification — the therapist.

In other words, Black Rhomb had used me as an object for externalizing her inner coflict. The struggle between us had been worked out as an external conflict about whether she could paint or not. She had persistently asserted that she could not paint at all — I had appealed to her latent talent.[2]

Notes to Discussion

1. Melanie Klein: The psychogenesis of manic-depressive states, pp. 306/307 (From *Contributions to Psycho-Analysis*, 1921 – 1945):

   "In the normal course of events the ego is faced at this point of its development — roughly between *four to five* months of age — with the necessity to acknowledge psychic reality as well as the external reality to a certain degree. It is thus made to realize that the loved object is at the same time the hated one; and, in addition to this, that the real objects and the real figures, both external and internal, are bound up with each other . . . both as *excessively good* and *excessively bad* figures, and that these two kinds of object relations intermingle and color each other to an ever increasing degree in the course of development. The first important steps in this direction occur, in my view, when the child comes to know its mother as a whole person and becomes *identified* with her as a whole, real loved person. It is then that the *depressive position* . . . comes to the fore." (My underlining.)

2. Anna Freud: *Normality and pathology in childhood* (1966), p. 42: The child analyst as object for externalization:

"The child thus restages his internal (intersystemic) conflicts as external battles with the analyst, a process which provides useful material. To interpret such externalizations in terms of object relationship within the transference would be a mistake . . . Understood in this manner, externalization is a sub-species of transference."

p. 233:
"Ego attitudes are changed where opportunities for identification are opened up, or superego pressure relieved by opportunity for suitable externalization."

4 Eagle

NARRATIVE

Eagle was 19 years old when she consulted me for her bulimia. Two years before this I had had her and her mother in therapy for six months, 30 session altogether, because of a difficult family situation.

Her present, all-consuming problem was her eating orgies. She was "listless, gloomy and brooding"; her eating problem was "disgusting," and she was guilt-ridden and felt especially "wicked towards mother." We agreed to try art-interpreting therapy, one session a week till the summer, that is, for about 6 months.

My ambitions for the first sessions were to find out which artistic medium was the most suitable — crayons, colored pencils, poster colors and brushes, or finger paint; in addition, I was hoping to obtain a pictorial expression of her relationship to internalized parental figures and self, of which up to this point I only had her verbal account.

In her first session I encourage her to draw her father. She does so, (Picture no. 1) using a brown pencil. The drawing resembles her father, slightly caricatured. It is a quickly drawn sketch. I ask about her associations to the picture:

"Square, benevolent."

Then I ask her to draw mother (Picture no. 2). In return I get *Mother in bed with migraine headache* — a motionless figure, covered by the bedspread, a sharp profile, closed eyes and long, yellow hair. A dark background emphasizes the gloomy atmosphere. Her drawing occupies only half of the sheet.

"Something is missing in the picture," I suggest.

Whereupon she draws "a wall" to the left of the bed, herself on the other side of the wall, rigid, gazing in the direciton of where her mother is lying.

"What comes to your mind?"

"It's myself behind a wall — hesitating to go in —"

"Anything else?"

"No."

I ask her to draw "mother a long time ago, the first Mommy."

She draws the torso and head of a woman — (Picture no. 3) — it is done "en face", with wide open, staring eyes; a wry smile, long, straight, yellow hair — a light green dress with red dots. Her association is that her father doesn't like the fact that Eagle is considering leaving home.[2] I show her the discrepancy between the staring eyes and the wry smile in her portrait; she dismisses this, however, claiming that it is purely accidental.

In her next session I ask her to draw herself. I get a picture that is quickly drawn, Picture no. 4. She says it is a fantasy-figure, she has drawn it before. Her association to it is "a bird of prey," later she refers to it as "the Eagle."

I think the picture holds both aggression and self-denigration. The aggressive part of it contains a ravenous element. The body is only hinted at, but appears to be swelling to an infinitely vast size.

"I think the discrepancy between the look of this sinister bird of prey and the way you look is quite remarkable! The only thing you have in common with the eagle is the watchful look in the eyes — I think, however, that you are using this portrait as an excuse to put yourself down."

She tells me that she has developed this self portrait over the last couple of years:

"It's supposed to be self-mocking, a bit tragic, and — a bit humorous. But the eagle's wickedness is not successfully rendered."

"How is that?"

"It wasn't supposed to be so stupid — this eagle isn't doing anything — isn't catching any lambs. It is probably trying to be a lone, predatory and independent eagle, one that follows its instincts, like a real eagle ..."

She interrupts herself:

"It's not the eagle's fault that she was born an eagle! That she flies higher than all the others, lives alone in her nest — reigning over the others with supreme authority and catching her prey as she wishes!"

She has gotten herself into quite a state, I think, building up a pile of self-accusations.

"Can you draw a different kind of bird, an 'anti-eagle'?"

Her reply is a picture of a red teddy-bear, (Picture no. 5), with meek eyes looking up into a light green cloud. She explains that it is supposed to be "a mixture of a teddy-bear and a pig, the kind of fantasy figure that little children make up."

"How is the piggy-bear feeling?"

"Like it was in a vacuum, all empty and grey — it's a feeling of uncertainty — and of something tragic and depressing."

The next session is spent going through the discrepancies between her self-portrait and her real appearance, and between the cuddly and the pig-like qualities she endowed the teddy-bear with. Her association here is that she remembers crying as a small girl, feeling worthless, mean and wicked, and picking up her baby brother [3] to comfort herself. And she remembers thinking that "mother was mean and unfair;" whereas she herself was the "just" one.

There is no more time for painting this session; a great deal of bitterness needs to be expressed.

I judge that the time is ripe for a decision on a suitable art medium and suggest fingerpaint the next session, thus hoping to by-pass Eagle's tendency to intellectualize. She is divided between her wish to try out the paint and her fear that she is going to betray herself. These conflicting feelings are revealed both verbally and through her paintings. First she paints "something round, like a whirl of paint, something is closed in, it's moving inwards, inwards —". It turns into a multi-colored whirl in the middle of the sheet (Picture no. 6), then she adds "something revolting, rigid and irrevocable." — the black and yellow vertical bars to the left of the picture. [4]

I try to make her associate to certain parts of the composition. First to the circle, starting with the green dots.

"This is candy."

"And the black stuff?"

"Something frightening."

She has no associations to the red and yellow areas in the center of the figure. The vertical bars stand for "shut off."

I praise her for the good composition and the clarity of her pictorial language:

"Precisely! This is why you're here, you feel shut off from the rest of society because of the perpetual, grinding whirlpool of over-eating and vomiting that you have gotten yourself into!"

She responds with another picture (Picture no. 7). It has a firm, symmetrical structure, except for the brown, studded base. Her associations to the symmetrical green and black areas are:

"It makes me feel split up, like being mad."

"I do not see any insanity here! It is controlled and strictly symmetrical, but what comes to your mind if you look at the brown base underneath?"

"That's the foundation![5]"

"What will become of this, then?"

She responds with Picture no. 8 and says:

"Everything is destroyed, messed up!"

The red, green and yellow lump of paint in the center is painted over with firm strokes of brown and brownish-black.

It is all going too smoothly for her now — it is becoming a little theatrical. I wish to point this out to her, and say in my fairy-tale voice:

"And then everything was all wrecked and gone ..."

I get a prompt response: she paints *Idyllic landscape* (Picture no. 9). The sun is shining from a clear blue sky on field flowers in a green meadow! She smiles sarcastically.

When it is time for her next appointment, I pick up on her feeling of being split and ask her to elaborate somewhat on the subject. With her fingers she paints a composition of vertical lines, broken up in the center by a narrow "inlet" (Picture no. 10). The first part of the sketch is done in black, then to the left she paints a green and a brown vertical line. This is repeated on the right-hand side, only here the brown line is replaced by a red one. Finally she fills in the narrow inlet with green and violet fingerprints, with red at the innermost part of the inlet. She uses the same technique on the right-hand side, in green this time.

As before, this is a symmetrical composition, this time with a central archaic symbol, the "inlet" or "entrance". (See Introduction, Archaic uterine symbols.) What comes to her mind is:

"Contact from two sides."

"That means you are in the middle?"

"Yes.[6]"

"I think the picture says that on one side you are experiencing pressure from your father, the brownish-green part. You painted him before, in brown. On the other side you feel pressurized by mother. Previously you painted her in a green dress with a red pattern. Please paint your relationship to mother."

She answers with Picture no. 11 and paints a narrow yellow inlet with broad strokes of the finger. She calls it *The receiving agency as seen from the back*. She fills in half of the opening with green paint. Next to it appears a brown line, finally "some black rubbish."

She says that the brown paint represents herself, the green is mother. The brown paint was physically *inserted* into the opening whereas the green paint seemed more like a coating or lining of the inner wall. I ask if anything is forcing its way into the "receiving agency".[7] Her response is another picture, where the black paint in the center arrives first (Picture no. 12). She is more engaged now, and her mood has changed — she is a little introspective. The black paint is laid on in swift, firm strokes, ending in arrows which are directed at the base. Finally a back-and-forth motion below the arrow heads, still in black, without taking the time to put more paint on her fingers. The black line is extended to enclose the arrows. Her association to this picture is:

"This is what gives me a bad conscience, the black part with the arrows is me, the embrace is my mother's."

I remind her of the back-and-forth movement:

"What does it represent?"

"Mother is lying down there, embracing me."

The picture has an archaic shape[8], and reflects a sadistic attack on the mother figure.

"It looks like you have protested a great deal against this embrace before!"

She arrives very late for her next session and asks if she may make up the lost time at the end of the session. This gives me an excellent opportunity to bring up the transference situation.

"Can you paint what it's like coming to the sessions?"

The picture consists of three parts — before, during and after a therapy session, from left to right (Picture no. 13). She begins by painting from the left grey, horizontal strokes, puts some traces of green in the grey field, continues in brilliant colors — white, light pink and a bright green which she obtains by mixing white into the green paint. It has a red center. A small amount of red is added at the base also. The whole thing is framed in blackish-brown paint, which she also uses for the continuation, horizontal, short, fiery strokes to the right of the frame. Calmer, brown, horizontal strokes take over, ending opposite the starting point. A premeditated composition.

Associating to "before the session", she says:

"The grey is the listlessness and the green is the anticipation."

To the part which represents "during the session" she adds:

"Something clear, brilliant, and balanced. — And then I have to frame it, put an end to it by locking the door, and all at once it's getting darker — and I'm out in the grey again."

I comment on the apparent contradiction between her arriving late and her wish to prolong the session.

"I think you enjoy coming here, while at the same time you find it difficult. Unconsciously you are holding back, by arriving late, but the clear, blue thoughts wish to prolong the session. The picture contains something of the same idea — coming here is "clear and balanced", but you have to put a thick frame around it and put the lock on the door?"

"I don't trust you! You influence me!"

"What does that remind you of?"

"Mother!"

We agree that she should come here twice a week for some time ahead.[9]

No reminders are necessary at the start of her next session. She spontaneously produces a large, arched shape "which presses down on me, black and heavy. (Picture no. 14). Underneath she put some short blue, green and yellow strokes of paint with some red mixed in.

"I *want* it to be like that, no matter what you say," she says.[10]

"But perhaps the heavy, black thing reminds you of something?"

"I dreamed that I came to Daddy's place, he lived in a red townhouse. There was a gloomy and tragic atmosphere there, and the houses were different from the ones at home. But Daddy wasn't there, I looked and looked for him, thinking he might be dead."

"What happened the day before?[11]"

"I spent the week-end with Daddy, and cried because he had to leave home, felt sorry for him, worried that something might happen to him."

I ask her to write down the dream, so we can discuss it later.

Next time I ask her to paint another self-portrait.[12] It turns into a variation of the eagle, (Picture no. 15.) This time she departs from the fantasy-figure, which was purely a bird of prey. The long, blackish-brown hair lends a human, feminine touch to the picture. The face, and especially the red mouth, still has a ravenous, preying expression. The body is shapeless, but it has a green and yellow spotted design. This may signify a positive, anticipating attitude — she has used the same technique earlier to symbolize such qualities. (See Picture no. 13.) Her style is now swinging from conscious naturalism to spontaneous non-figurative symbolism. Her comment on the picture:

"Diffuse, that's all I can say."

"We have to make it clearer!"

I wish to find out what "the heavy, black thing that presses down on me" signifies, and say:

"If that heavy, black something didn't press down on you, then what? Can you paint that?"

She responds with a naturalistic painting, Picture no. 16.

"A sturdy tree which is firmly rooted," she says.

She paints red and green fruit on it, some "fall to the ground." I take it to be a projection of her wish to be creative, and leave it at that.

"You said earlier that I exert an influence over you, while at the same time you associated this to mother. Can you paint that?"

This time I obtain a response which has a totally different composition (Picture no. 17). First she paints a vigorous, black circle at the lower right-hand corner of the sheet. She fills in the circle with bright yellow paint. Outside the circle, to the left, she paints "speed-stripes" in violet and green paint, which creates an illusion of movement downwards to the right. A violet line is penetrating a barely indicated opening in the black circle. I describe the picture graphically/expressionistically as I see it. Her comment:

"An egg that is fertilized from behind."

"What does it mean, 'from behind'?"[13]

But she has no immediate reply.

The next time she comes, I ask for the notes from the dream

about father and the red houses. She doesn't have any. I encourage her to try painting some of the remembered scenes from parts of the dream[14], starting with "arriving at Daddy's, who lived in a red town-house."

It turns into a couple of red rectangles, (Picture no. 18,) and a brown road, which keeps dividing.

"I couldn't find him — ... but this isn't the way it was!"

She pushes the painting aside. I encourage her to associate freely to a new picture, and *Sitting behind a yellow window, looking out* arrives (Picture no. 19). This is a naturalistic painting — a brightly yellow window frame and green and blue scenery outside, with a black area shaped like a mountain. Her association:

"I remember when I was about 10 years old, mother and I were together constantly. She was very strict and made all the decisions — I wasn't allowed to have my hair cut or go out — I spent my time reading magazines, eating tomato sandwiches — it was so dull, I wanted to take my own life."

"Perhaps you were a little angry too?"

The next time she resolutely starts on another picture: *Poorly disguised anger*! (Picture no. 20). It is a circular, brightly colored picture with a bright, red center. I follow her with graphic comments as she goes along. Dark-red and black stripes radiate from the center, which is surrounded by a fat, blue circle. Finally she breaks up the radiation with some red lines, which she puts in the outer part of the radiation field with some circular movements of her finger. The result is both a nucleus radiating power and a circular prohibitive agent. She has no additional comments on the picture.

"You said 'poorly disguised anger,' still it looks like you are managing to subdue your anger fairly well!"

I point to the clear blue circle around the center:

"It's quite substantial, as if clear, blue thoughts are restricting the vehement feelings. And as if this isn't enough, you try to stop some of the red and black beams by breaking them up with the red, circular strokes!"

She answers quite angrily:

"Anybody with the slightest ability to think clearly ..."

(She obviously wants to attack me for "the clear, blue thoughts.")

"Yes, what about them? Will they be punished?"

She is finally going somewhere and paints: *Angry*! (Picture no. 21).

"... it's almost all black, square, occupying almost the whole sheet ... a small, yellow, shining center ..." I comment as she goes along. She smiles as she puts down the small yellow center and says:

"As long as there is life, there is hope!"

I think she means that the black, punishing element is quite overwhelming, but that she spots an opening, and I say:

"I think that you almost condemned yourself, or thought that I condemned you, to death, eternal darkness!"

She paints her last picture this session: To the left "an egg with a yellow yolk," meaning: "to be in clover." To the right is "a withered orchid, perhaps something from the outside did it, exhaust, perhaps?"

"Well, if it was, it must have been your own exhaust!"

It is obvious that she is relating the punishment of her anger to an external factor.

During the following session I try to guide her towards her relationship to her internalized father figure, and encourage her to paint this. She paints two versions: First a multicolored composition to the left, (Picture no. 23,) she calls it, "connection with a fixed frame." "The frame" is the two vertical bars, "the connection" is the multicolored horizontal stripes in red, green, black, yellow, blue and white. The other version is in two colors, brown and white. The composition is now standing on its edge, with the frame in brown and the connecting part in white.

"What comes to your mind when you look at this fixed frame?"

She paints on another sheet, (Picture no. 24): *Daddy's apartment — we have a practical relationship*. And she paints, while I comment, "a naturalistic picture with a sofa, a table and lots of good food and TV." I ask her if there are other possibilities, relations on a different level — and she paints, in the same colors, a non-figurative composition, Picture no. 25. Her association is:

"It's tight and compact, over-protecting, and secure, bordering on dull."

"Anything else?"

Upon which she produces Picture no. 26 in clear pastels, a light and airy composition:

"Aesthetically comfortable, like the therapy-sessions — it stands for something good, the real me!"

"What about the compact aspect?"

The answer is a square composition in green and brown, picture no. 27, an irregular nucleus painted in raw sienna, surrounded by a green square. She says,

"Still more infiltrated, lifeless, and immobile (*the brown field*), loathsome and suffocatingly embracing, (*the green area*.)"

In her next session I try to interpret the most recent pictures for her while referring to earlier pictures:

"I think you have loved your father very much."

"He gave me the most attention, I was his pet. My older brother was always jealous."

"But at the same time you were envious of your father, you wished you could take his place — and get rid of him! In your dream you couldn't find him and you thought he was dead."

"In my dream wicked people had abducted him and killed him — not me."

"But it was *your* dream!" And I add:

"In the pictures of your relationship to your father and me, it was necessary to secure everything within a solid frame. Perhaps the solid frame reflected your wish to have something to hold on to — for ever?" I refer to the picture of *The receiving agency*,

"where the brown paint, which is you, is forcing its way into the 'receiving agency'."

Referring to Picture no. 12, "with the dangerous black arrows" which are pointing at mother who is lying underneath:

"You said there was some black rubbish in the receiving-agency. I think you wanted to eliminate it. But at the same time you worried that you yourself might be eliminated?"

"That makes me so mad!"

"Can you paint that?"

She responds with Picture no. 28: *Disgusting*!. The frame is in reddish-brown, inside is a violet rectangle. A diagonal bar, "locked at both ends," divides the picture. Her only comment is:

"Disgusting!"

"I think it looks like a frame that you have reinforced with a solid beam. In other words, you're saying: Enough is enough! And then you put a lock and bar on this subject!"

She responds by painting "a yellow tree that reaches out, but is intercepted by mother" (black).

"Is this an act of revenge?"

"U-humm." (Picture no. 29).

The following session, in order to catch any reactions, I encourage her to paint whatever comes to her mind. This turns out to be a self-portrait in two versions, first a humorous one to the right, then a variation and elaboration of the eagle-portrait to the left (Picture no. 30).

"The eagle is getting more human all the time," is my comment. Her comment: "a punk."

Obviously this is as far as she wishes to elaborate on the subject, because from now on she just wants to joke or talk about practical things, get my advice. But she continues to paint, first a painting of flowers and a black cloud, (Picture no. 31), then "a blue house with trees and a sun" — conventional and diversionary. (Picture no. 32). Finally two abstract compositions, which are both talented and decorative. (Pictures no. 33 and 34.)

We have two more sessions before, for practical reasons, we have to terminate the therapy, and I wish to consolidate what we have achieved. In her next session, therefore, I ask her to pick up again on her relationship to me. This develops into a composition where a group of stripes of different colors, (herself), are spinning around freely, but at the same time is fastened to something (Picture no. 35). She accentuates the ambiguity of the composition by attaching the spinning part to a green rack. Her association:

"I feel like a cloud with ties that are fastened to the ground — finally!"

"Then perhaps you could try to express your relationship to father again, too?"

It turns into a symmetrical composition (Picture no. 36), in white, blue and green. Her comment:

"A kind of unification of previous arguments, reminds me of a girl's crotch, but not in an indecent way.[15]" The green and the blue fans out and the opening is filled in with white paint. The brush strokes go down towards the point of unification.

"The picture seems to express reconciliation."

Finally:

"Can you please re-state your relationship with mother?"

She makes two versions. First a composition which she immediately says is a failure, and which she will not comment on. Then *The cloth-ball*, the shape of a ball, (Picture no. 37), made up of fields of various colors, with yellow, green and blue as the main colors.

The yellow and green fields are confined by some relatively thin black lines. In addition the bottom of the ball is colored violet. About the picture she says:

"Many good, separate things are squeezed together here, sometimes poorly so, and this gets worse because the black paint is squeezed in between the fields."

For the first time she tells me, in her abrupt manner, and with a wry smile:

"I was supposed to have been aborted. Mother went into hospital to have an abortion, but somebody convinced her not to, or she changed her mind, I don't know."

"That explains why there is an element of black between you, doesn't it? But there seems to be less of it now."

In her last session I want her to clarify what she has called "the receiving agency," her description of the archaic symbol which has run through the whole of this therapy.

"Can you paint 'a giving agency,' the opposite of a 'receiving agency'?"

"Mother's or my own?"

"Both.[16]"

Hesitatingly, she paints a sketch. (Picture no. 38). The composition is broken up into four parts: an elongated, brown triangle, a green ball, a blue rod and finally what she herself calls "the original giving agency," a yellow corn-stock, turned upside-down.

"It is giving because it is open."

"But the opening turns downwards — don't the contents run out?"

"Around this place you don't get anything free of charge, do you?" she says in a good-natured voice.

"You're right, that's the way it is around here![17]"

I point to the fact that there is no connection between the blue, green and red shapes:

"Can you make this composition more unified?"

Whereupon she paints a centered composition within a brown frame, divided into four parts by two diagonal lines. (Picture no. 39). In one of the resulting sections she paints herself, an all white field. This is supposed to represent the fact that she is viewing herself from outside. I interpret it to be a sign that she feels able to accept things from outside (other people), but not too successful when it comes to receiving things from within the square, (her family).

"What was it like before, a long, long time ago?"

Another picture, no. 40. A light green circular area in the middle is surrounded by a ring of sweets.

"This is me, in the middle, the first me, with all sorts of colors around me."

"Yes, that's what it's like being a baby, you receive care all the time. Actually this has turned into a receiving agency."

She chooses another sheet of paper and quickly paints picture no. 41, a black vertical line, and a green disc on each side of the line.

"This one isn't getting anything."

She paints the left disc black.

"And this one is getting too much! (*She fills the 'dish' with 'sweets'*). Too much or too little, it's all just as bad."

"You said this situation is splitting you up. Now I see what you mean."

"U-humm."

She paints a wide, smiling mouth at the bottom of the page and laughs at the effect:

"It looks like a face with an evil eye and a green eye filled with sweets, and in the middle a long nose!" (In the sense of getting nothing out of it.)

A year later Eagle contacted me again to ask my advice concerning choice of jobs. She told me that her problem of bulimia was over. She had short spells of over-eating now and then, but these were getting less and less frequent. Her over-eating was now consciously controlled.

Notes to Narrative

1. The family treatment had consisted of therapy sessions with Eagle and her mother, both individually and together, and sporadic conversations with both parents and Eagle.
2. Her father, who has moved out of the home, is worried how her mother will manage without Eagle.
3. She has two brothers, one is three years older and one is nine years younger.
4. One of the themes in this symbolic composition is the same as in the picture *Mother in bed with a migraine headache* (Picture no. 2.): the theme being " my unapproachable mother." In addition this composition symbolizes her bulimia, (the grinding, circular element,) and how it isolates her from the outside world. (The vertical bar.) This theme is repeated in a later picture as well, *The big, black square with the bright, longed for, yellow center*. (Picture no. 21.) The theme is an expression of a central conflict in her relationship to her internal mother-figure.
5. I think she is moving on two levels simultaneously, both in this picture and the previous one: (a) Her problem with bulimia, (b) her relationship to mother. In the picture with the grinding whirl in the center and the two vertical bars on the left-hand side, (Picture no. 6), the yellow and reddish-brown in the center of the whirl stand for the internalized mother shutting herself off and Eagle's hatred. The vertical bars in black and yellow represent her ambivalent feelings towards mother — the yellow being her longing for contact, the black being the punishment for the negative feelings she is harboring. This picture reflects the attempts of her inner censoring agent to repress and disguise her infantile impulses. In the picture with the symmetric, "splitting" composition on a brown pedestal, or base, (Picture no. 7,) she is expressing her fear that she will become insane as a result of the double pressure; the pressure from mother and from herself. On the other hand, it could represent Eagle's bearing down on mother to "make her even with the ground" or to force her into a state of insanity. This would turn her into an intolerable instrument of sadistic torture, which her superego could

not accept. The pedestal may be, as she herself puts it, "a stand or a foundation." She obviously wants to display something, and it might be this gruesome, infantile impulse that she is "putting on the stand."

Freud, on referring to the work of condensation in the production of dreams: "The manifest dream is short, scanty, and laconic compared to the profuseness of the dream thoughts." (S. Freud: Drommetydning," Part II, p. 8).

6. I find it difficult to advance at this point, I do not know which level she is on. Physically she finds herself in a difficult position between her parents who have separated, but who still stick together in some respects. There is also the possibility that she is on an intra-psychic level, that the opposing agencies in her relationship to her mother are exerting pressure on her in several ways. The only certain clue which can help us to move further is the fact that she has previously drawn her father in brown and painted her mother in red and green.

7. In my comments here, I rely on the movement of the hand and the direction of the brush-strokes.

8. All three pictures in this session have a central, archaic form, "the inlet" in the picture with "contact from both sides," (Picture no. 10), "the receiving agency" in Picture no. 11, and the circular "embrace" in Picture no. 12. Margaret Naumburg refers to such forms in her book, *An Introduction to Art Therapy*, and says: "The use of archetypal uterine-symbols attempts to express intimate feelings about sexuality, moods or changes within oneself."

Regarding the visual, revived images on which dreams are based, Sigmund Freud writes: "(These) also display a number of archaic characteristics, such as the use of a symbolism (in this case of a predominantly sexual kind) which it has since also been possible to discover in other spheres of mental activity."

These are the first of Eagle's pictures to have the characteristics of a dream. Symbolically the "inlet", "the receiving agency," and "the embrace" represent the uterus in the archaic language of form. The pictures symbolize her sadistic assaults on her mother's womb.

9. I wish to see her twice a week since she is now trying to sort out her relationship to her internalized mother figure, which is extremely complicated and abounding with contradictions, and because I need a strong transference relationship to handle the negative transference; if not, I would risk a break in the therapy.
10. This is an angry and obstinate comment which she expects me to cut short, the way her mother would. The negative transference is escalating.
11. I am trying to find out what triggered the dream — what happened the day before she dreamt it.
12. My intention is to direct her towards the transference situation through the self portrait.
13. This composition is not accidental. Previously she has painted a "cave" or "inlet", now she is painting "an egg." The first two represent archaic uterine-symbols, the last one alludes to fertilization in the uterus.

She has not supplied any material which would explain what "from behind" stands for — it may reflect an infantile impulse to usurp her mother's place with father, or deprive her of her childbearing potential. Or it may stand for a paranoid, backbiting element that she belives herself to be influenced by.

14. When using dreams, as in the analysis of dream-related pictures, it is of vital importance that one obtains associations/pictorial responses to the individual elements of the manifest dream/projected picture. In this case the material needed is missing.
15. Picture no. 36 is a pictorial response directed at reconciliation with the father, both verbally, (her comment on the picture,) and figuratively. Margaret Naumburg, in *An Introduction to Art Therapy*, gives several examples of such symmetric color-compositions as expressions of the "unification of two opposing aspects — symmetrical balance." "The crotch of a girl, but not in an indecent way," I interpreted (like herself?) as a reminiscence of the oedipal situation. (See the white paint.)
16. I leave it to her to decide whether she is going to paint this together or separately. She is here displaying her

continuing problems in distinguishing between which is herself and which is her mother in her mind. ("mother's or my own?)

By using the expression, "the giving agency" I follow her own terminology; by inquiring after the opposite of "the receiving agency" I try to help her gain the kind of insight which is made possible through the introduction of an opposite element.

17. I think her remark has a double meaning: "You are frustrating me," and "New insight is paid for in pain." Therefore my remark: "Yes, that's how it is."

DISCUSSION

DIAGNOSTIC

Eagle was 19 years of age and for several years she had had persistent symptoms of bulimia with compulsive food orgies for longer periods of time, but without signs of anorexia. Her voracious appetite seemed closely tied to an ambivalent fixation on her internalized mother figure. But she had retained a certain measure of protest, even revolt (e.g. she moved out of her parents' home), which is an indication that the masochistic element had not taken over yet. On the other hand, she showed distinct signs of depression and had arrived at a standstill in her work and as far as her further education was concerned. Her resources were to be found in her good general functioning, her artistic talent and her ability to get back on her feet again in times of trouble.

THERAPEUTIC GOAL

A certain measure of emancipation and struggle for independence had been in effect after the family therapy two years earlier, but her symptoms of bulimia were unchanged. The therapeutic goal was therefore to relieve her as much as possible of her infantile fixations so that she would be able to relinquish, or at least control, her food orgies.

BEYOND WORDS

THERAPEUTIC METHOD

We had half a year at our disposal, that is, about 20 weekly sessions. I chose the art interpreting form of therapy with fingerpaint as a means of communication.

Many of the pictures in this therapy are "prompted" pictures. Often this is true only of the first picture of the session, however. I chose this guided form of art interpretation therapy because I already have a thorough knowledge of her problems, and therefore may assume that this will strengthen rather than interfere with the therapy process, and because our time is limited.

One of Eagle's resources was her artistic talent. The method was therefore well suited to her, in one respect, but the danger of "artification" was also present, i.e. that she might want to create interesting and talented pictures to ward off spontaneous pictures containing unconscious and pre-conscious material.

Among her other resources were good schooling and verbal fluency — a talent which might tempt her to try to use intellectualization as a means of avoidance, but which also might enable her to transfer the beneficial effect of the therapy to other areas of her life such as her personal life, work and education.

The main, underlying problem was her depression. Would this guided form of therapy only serve to increase her intellectual insight while intensifying the depression? Against this I only had my confidence in the power of this method, through the pictorial creativity it demands, — to ensure an emotional reliving of the issues.

In the first four sessions I try to encourage a heightened experience of the relationship to her internalized father and mother figure through portraits and self-portraits, and help her clarify and live through the self-portrait.

In her fifth session she spontaneously presents the maelstrom, or grinding whirl in which she finds herself, of which the bulimia is an expression. She sees a connection between this and the isolation from the outside world which she is so acutely aware of.

Shortly afterwards she paints a picture which symbolizes the oral aggression which threatens to split her up and drive her towards insanity.

The symbolic expressions she is projecting are strong and clear. It seems as though the method is helping her to avoid the pitfall of intellectualizing her problems.

In her sixth session she paints two archiaic pictures; the first is "the receiving agency" (Picture no. 11) which, exceedingly condensed, symbolizes her jealousy and the oedipal conflict. The sadistic assault on her mother's womb, the first manifestation of her jealousy, is the central theme and is responsible for the mythical and abstract character of the picture.

A somewhat simpler presentation is the picture with the dark, aggressive darts pointing at the mother figure and the mother's embrace, (Picture no. 12), where she displays her protest against the clinging care that the mother figure is providing, and which is impeding Eagle's struggle towards individualisation.

The transference situation is treated in her seventh session, Picture no. 13, on a pre-conscious level. The situation develops into a mother-transference, the way we see it for example in Picture no. 17; the influence of mother and the therapist become one and the same in the picture and is symbolized by an "egg which is fertilized from behind." This is probably experienced as a reactionary influence and triggers a sub-paranoid attitude.

The transference situation develops further. In her 11th session (Picture no. 21) she paints *Being angry*: the black square with the bright yellow center. It is an aggressive picture which (a) is aimed at me as a mother figure, (b) represents a punishing aggression towards self, and (c) portrays a dawning hope that she will be able to reach mother. The mode of communication, the artistic picture, makes possible the expression of the many voices in a particularly beautiful way and extends the breadth of the therapeutic effect. I especially emphasize the self-punishing aspect in the picture because I think this issue requires most attention at this point.

If we follow the transference situation on to her 15th session, Picture no. 35, where it is painted and described as "free, but dependent" we see that she has made a leap forwards towards independence and realistic insight. The three archaic pictures (*The receiving agency*, Picture no. 11, *The embrace*, Picture no. 12, and *The egg*, Picture no. 17) are especially interesting, (a) because they show the depth of the fixation, (b) because they show how closely it is tied to her relationship to an internalized mother figure, (c) because they show how sibling rivalry and oedipal conflict complicate the situation.

I think the creative production of these pictures, the pictorial and verbal associations she produced in connection with them, and the therapeutic interpretations I could offer were essential elements in this therapy. The externalization of the hating and self destructive elements were particularly well presented in Picture no. 12, "the black darts aimed at Mommy's body and the motherly embrace", Picture no. 20, *Poorly disguised anger*; Picture no. 21 *Being angry*, and Picture no. 25, *Disgusting*. The effect of this form of transference has played an important part in attaining the favorable result that was the outcome of this therapy.

The reconciliation showed itself towards the end of the therapy, in Picture no. 36, *The not indecent girl's crotch*, in relation to the father figure; Picture no. 37, *The cloth ball* in relation to the mother figure.

The final part of the therapy was spent working through the issues again.

The result after one year proves that the attempt to help her gain sufficient control over her problem with bulimia was successful.

5 Punishing Iron

NARRATIVE

Punishing Iron had ceased to develop normally from the time he was two years of age. As time went by, he demonstrated symptoms that clearly pointed to an autistic psychotic development, and his parents described him as a restless boy, difficult to reach — health personnel described him as a boy with an atypical development and poorly developed language distinguished by echolalia, neologisms and a lack of personal pronouns. His anxiety was of an archaic type, described as "doomsday-anxiety". Under the assumption that he was suffering from a central nervous dysfunction with autistic traits which had affected his speech center, he had had special education from 5 to 12 years of age.

When he was 13 years old, I, inspired by his music therapists, suggested to his parents that he should begin weekly art-interpretation therapy, which they agreed to. This would obviously have to be a long-term project, 4 years at least. I will describe the first phase of the treatment.[1]

ESTABLISHING A CHANNEL OF COMMUNICATION
THROUGH CRAYONS AND FAIRY-TALES.

The first three months of therapy consisted of my reading fairy-tales aloud while he drew, using crayons. By reading fairy-tales aloud I hoped to establish a channel of communication.[2] During the first few sessions I read from the fairy-tales of the Brothers Grimm in an even, monotonous voice with my face partly turned away from him, as if I was just reading out into the air. I did not attempt to make contact with him beyond reading aloud. He slowly grew accustomed to the therapy room and accepted the fact that he was supposed to sit at the desk and draw. When he drew, he exerted a lot of pressure on the crayon, and mostly drew 4-5 cm long stripes in various colors. (Picture no. 1). He was silent, except for abrupt statements like "Want juice!" or tentative remarks like: "Irons — twice as hot as the hottest thing in the world?" Sometimes he would utter ominous statements like "Jaws!" (Referring to the movie about the shark which attacked people on a beach,) or "Am crazy!"

Often he would sit for long periods just scraping wax off the crayons with his finger nails.[3]

After three or four sessions I began to modulate my voice somewhat. Every time the story conveyed oral aggression, I put on a dramatic expression while gradually raising my voice. I did this with increasing intensity. The most dramatic episodes were read over and over. Presently he began to react in response to the expressions on my face. He began to press down even harder while drawing his patterns of lines. Eventually he began to cover one colored line with another. This was done in an exceedingly aggressive manner when the violent part of the story grew near its climax. We were finally able to communicate![4]

I did not fully understand what this aggressive method of covering up lines stood for, but was fairly convinced that it stood for something fundamental and annihilating. I also observed that he would still revert spontaneously to his habit of scraping wax off the crayons — an activity which rendered him psychotically inaccessible.

FINGER-PAINTING

I therefore decided on another, softer medium, finger-paint.[5] I was now able to discontinue my practice of reading Grimm's fairy-tales aloud — the special dramatic quality of these stories had had the desired effect — and I began to describe to him graphically his artistic efforts down to the minutest detail. (See Introduction, Graphic Clarification.)

Annihilation through finger-painting.
In the period that followed, I discovered why he covered up lines with a new layer of color — he wanted to annihilate the underlying color! (Picture no. 2). Often he would increase the destructive effect by scraping the picture with his nail. I began to dramatize this, following up his actions with a graphic clarification. Drama followed drama, on each occasion climaxing just in time before he was able to annihilate a colored line or shape.

The first direct attack.
I began to use voice-modulation again, to dramatize my choice of words and body-language. When we reached the point where he was about to annihilate his design, I stopped him and he uttered the first statement that was aimed directly at me: "Kill you!" I said: "I know that," and praised him for the clarity of his statement. He had never used the word "you" correctly before.

After three months he mastered this painting "routine," and allowed me to stop him before he was able to annihilate his design. Throughout this period his art was strictly non-figurative.

POSTER-COLORS

Around the time that he was able to refrain from annihilating his designs, I gave him poster-colors and withdrew the fingerpaint — partly because it tended to get very messy, and partly because I wanted him to express himself more accurately — something which might be easier with a brush. I also wanted to offer him the possibility of emotional distance. This would be especially important if the content and extension of the destructive element in his artistic endeavours should become clear to him at some time in the future. So far, this was not a problem, since psychologically speaking he was not yet a person.

Identifying the colors.
In the two months that followed, I encouraged him to identify the colors (Picture no. 3, dated 28 May and no. 4, dated 10 June). On referring to these pictures, he increasingly maintains that: BLUE stands for food, or "yum-yum"; RED stands for danger, strength, something red-hot, for instance "twice as hot as the hottest thing in the world"; dark GREY-GREEN and BROWN stand for something that spills all over, or the result of red being permitted to destroy, for instance, blue. Finally, YELLOW has to go with "penis" or 'urinating."

Once in a while he would depart from this color scheme, but the main trend was clear at this point. Later on he changed his color scheme and also added to it.

Symbolic use of colors.
In his third picture on 28 May he creates a distinct sequence: first he paints a yellow, arched shape with an opening on the right-hand side (Picture no. 5), then a blue triangle which threatens to invade the yellow form from within. (He is easily stopped now, I only have to place my hand over his.) A red half-circle nearly encloses the yellow arch. As an alternative to annihilation, he is allowed to blend the three colors carefully, and the result is the dark blue-green round patch of color to the left.

The colors consume one another!
I describe the picture to him: "If blue is allowed to devour yellow, or yellow devours blue, then red will come and devour blue-yellow, and then ... (pointing to the dark blue-green patch,) everything will be destroyed, devoured!"[6]

In four pictures dated 10 June, 2 weeks later, he repeats this theme and the issue is still consumption or annihilation. In the first picture (Picture no. 6), he paints first of all the central blue circle, then the red shape which partly encloses the blue on the left. Then comes a similar yellow shape to the right. The dark, dirty-green patches appear while he is, with my permission, carefully blending the colors. While this is going on he is rocking his body, snorting and he appears to be sexually stimulated. He says,

"Love being 'græv'!" an expression he invents on the spot, a neologism. The word 'græv' resembles the Norwegian word "grov", meaning gross, obscene. Judging from his expression, the word seems to signify gleeful destruction.

Confused and afraid, not 'crazy'.
The time is three months later. We are back on the same trail; this time, however, events take place on a more conscious level. He has perceived what the word 'confused' stands for. The following is an illustration of this: When he shakes his head and says "don't know," but would prefer to have said "am crazy," he really means to say "confused." I have introduced the term 'confused' to him and have consistently rejected "am crazy," which until now he had used to provoke other people and enhance his own anxiety. He understood this peculiar way of

describing the term 'confused', so there was no reason for me to correct it. It helped prevent him from escaping into his psychosis.

On 2 September, I begin our session as follows:

"You are frightened and confused when one color devours another! Can you paint that?"[7]

He answers me with Picture no. 7. He starts out by putting blue, red and orange paint on the paper and proceeds to blend them carefully, under my supervision:

"Just so they don't devour each other!"

I give a pictorial description as he is proceeding and interpret it:

"All this is, is a whole new color, but you see destruction and punishment, and then you get confused. Can you make that even clearer?"

The Iron.
He paints the same thing (Picture no. 8), but adds with a ballpoint-pen a shape that is supposed to represent an iron.[8] He makes two of them on the left half of the sheet. One is partly filled in with "confused-colored" grey-green paint. "I think you are saying that confusion and iron is the same thing!" (The "confused", grey-green color is now of a brighter tone value. It will change into a brilliant value in Picture no. 19 where the color stands for himself *inside* the yellow "mother-color".)

A second direct attack.
In the next picture (Picture no. 9), he shows in the same manner that grey-green confusion also stands for my trousers. (I am wearing trousers of the same color.) Quick as lightning he turns to me and paints my trousers. "I think you are afraid that I will punish you if you let one color devour another!"

With the same speed as before, he puts two more brush-strokes on my trousers.

Magic protection.
In his 8th picture this session he introduces a new element: the magic X'es. (Picture no. 10). After he has gone through the procedure of near-devouring over and over, he quickly marks

the sheet with a couple of X'es. I offer the following explanation: "X stands for: don't devour! — Then you can be safe."

The Evil Companion.
Four weeks later a newcomer makes his entrance into our sessions. It turns out, however, that even if the eerie figure is new to me, his parents and teacher are already well acquainted with him. (Picture no. 11). The newcomer has a human trunk with arms and neck. But a grim, black symbol replaces the head. The symbol resembles two cymbals turned away from each other, connecting at the upper end of the neck.

I still represent punishment.
He writes DU (meaning "YOU") above the creature, and I take this to mean that in his mind, I have become synonymous with his evil companion. "You are afraid that I will punish you like the evil one!"[9]

The evil companion has an incomplete body. On his right leg is superimposed some unidentifiable scribble. The left leg becomes a thin line only, however, this could also symbolize a penis. (See Picture no. 12, which his teacher handed me. He had drawn it once when he was by himself, a few months earlier.)

To devour and be devoured!
One month later he has identified a blue patch as "boob," (Picture no. 13), a round, yellow shape, as "mouth." The mouth threatens to devour the breast, whereupon the mouth turns into the dusty-green field in the upper left-hand corner. "The punishment for devouring a breast is to be devoured," is my conclusion.

The punishing iron in the stomach has the power to annihilate.
Two months later we are still working on the same problem, with the punishing element gradually becoming a part of him. On 14 November he paints Picture no. 14. Here again we have the same colors, red, blue and yellow, threatening to devour each other. He does not have to blend the colors any more to get the desired hue — he keeps some pre-mixed paint in a jar! The

grey-green paint is not as dark and threatening as it was in the beginning.

When asked to associate to "devouring" today, he makes up a long tale. The gist of the story is that "one person attacks another," ("the other" probably being himself.) I try to cheer him up:

"I'm sure you are able to protect yourself!" which makes him fear that he'll get an iron in his stomach. I repeat,

"I know you can protect yourself!" whereupon he admits that he'll "heat ... (the aggressor) to 2 300°C!"

The Punishing Iron.
After this episode we begin to call the punishing element the Punishing Iron. (In other words, the cruel super-ego.) The magic X'es have a different function all of a sudden: From now on he uses them to magically prolong the session, that is, when I prepare him for the fact that the session is almost over, he swiftly puts an X on the sheet of paper.

Around this time the evil companion ceases to be synonymous with punishment (Picture no. 15). In this picture from 14 November he has, while we "talk" about punishment, drawn his companion with a pencil and colored him. He has furnished him with a blue trunk, the rest of the body is dirty-yellow, and the evil head-symbol is still black. But it is the first time he has been able to spend so much time with this figure, doing his job so carefully, without showing open anxiety.

Destruction of uterus, appropriating the content.
Two weeks later he picks up a picture he made the previous week and places a red patch inside what was supposed to be a mother-symbol (Picture no. 16). I ask him what came to his mind.

"If talk about it, what will I become then?" (He now uses the pronoun "I" about himself, temporarily?)

"No longer afraid that you are going to be devoured, or disappear!"

Then he paints three versions of this motif where red attacks the cerulean blue mother-symbol, whereupon he attacks it with his finger-nail, that is, he scrapes the paint out of the symbol. (Picture no. 17, dated 28 Nov.)

"Red is you?"
"M,m."

Beginning of symbiotic phase.
The next session he leans back towards me and wants me to sit close to him and hold him while he paints. He just wants to paint today.

"No talk today — want no talk today!"
"That's right, little babies don't talk —"

He paints light blue balls, (Picture no. 18), none of them aggressive.

Bubbly happy!
Next session brings more bubbles. He says that the balls are "bubble-happy."

For another month or so he paints happy bubbles, eating cookies, drinking juice and making sure I am sitting right behind him while he is painting.

All of a sudden the colors begin to attack one another again, and we get more rounds where I have to prevent him from killing and devouring!

Chasing Daddy out of Mommy
On 30 January I begin to talk about the boundaries that separate him from me — partly through the use of puppets, partly through referring to his pictures — where the content is Baby-Mommy during the process of individuation. His first graphic response to this is Picture no. 19. Here he has painted a Mommy-symbol with a light green-yellow center and he himself in the middle, that is, painted over like a turquoise nucleus in the middle of the Mommy symbol. Close by, on the right, is the Daddy-symbol as a red, rounded shape. He paints three versions of this while I describe the pictorial content.

In the third picture of this kind it suddenly strikes him:

"Eaten Mommy!" Whereupon turquoise invades yellow. He resolutely dumps the pens and pencils out of the mug on to the desk. [10] Then he assaults a fresh sheet with *Blue chasing red out of yellow* (Picture no. 20).

What he calls "blue" is really turquoise, that is, the symbol of himself; red has for a long time represented Daddy (or himself), and the dirty-yellow is Mommy. It is obvious that the turquoise "ball" with a brown point invades "Daddy," the red field in the middle, which again invades the cluster of pale grey-yellow circles. He says,

"Chasing Daddy out of Mommy — going crazy!"

The Punishing Iron is ejected.
The next session he is all grunting and retching, right from the beginning. I ask him what is bothering him.

"Throw up iron!" I hold out my hands to "receive" it. He coos and mimes that he is feeling better now. This scene is repeated over and over.[11]

Fear of castration.
While throwing up the iron into my hands, he is holding his own hands in front of his groin, like a warrior who fears castration, and I encourage him to go and check if his penis is still there. He does this, whereupon he nods gravely.[12]

For several sessions now, the main theme is the iron in Mommy's stomach. The iron is also in his own stomach, a punishment for having devoured a part of Mommy. He curls up close to me, feeling safe, and alternates between grinning and miming "crazy". The retaliation aspect is worked through and the same procedure is repeated over and over: He will express symbolically, by painting, his impulse to devour a part of Mommy. For this, he is punished by the iron inside him. He tries to project the iron, placing it into Mommy's body/me — and I say that I will keep it for him.

Temporary relapse.
The next session the problem is reactivated. He has been told that Mommy is going to have another baby. He tells me about it in telegraph-style:

"Mommy, new baby," and draws a naturalistic iron with the number 2 000 (degrees) next to it (Picture no 21). This turns out to be the last time for a while that we are able to go through this theme.

New learning.
Towards the end of the month he is eager to learn about the

colors of the rainbow (Picture no. 22). In this picture he is interrupted in his work (red, orange, yellow). He is distracted by a constructionwork of sticks which he has just made — he wants to copy it on the paper. The sticks are glued together with small lumps of modelling wax to form a comple structure.[13]

Distinguishing between himself and me.
In this period he is mainly preoccupied with learning new things. On 17 April he draws a presentation of himself and me (Picture no. 23). The composition consists of two ovals which slant somewhat — each with a dot placed in the center. They are drawn in soft pencil-lines, and between the ovals he places another line, more delicate still, and then the symbol of the evil one, next to us (the ovals.) He probably includes the symbol to challenge me, in a last effort to frighten me. The main thing, however, is that this is the first clear projection of his experience of being a person separated from me.

Separating outer from inner aggression.
About a month later, while presenting "something angry" in the shape of a black spot in the lower right-hand corner of the sheet (Picture no. 24), I ask him to define what kind of "angry" he is referring to. He says "angry" and points to himself.
  "What do other kinds of 'angry' look like, then?"
  He draws the three black, vigorous arrows aimed at the three circles and says:
  "You are all angry with me![14]"
  I praise him for being able to discriminate between his own anger and that of others. But I also take this to be an expression of his anger and worry that I should be angry with him, since we, for external reasons, will have to interrupt the therapy for a longer period of time. I tell him that it is OK to be angry, and assure him that the music-therapists are going to continue their work with him. Finally I ask him to draw the two of us. Quickly he jots down a presentation of himself, first, in the music-sessions (Picture no. 25), and then a picture of himself in my sessions (Picture no. 26). For the first time, he has projected himself as a person in his own right.

Notes to Narrative

1. At the time of writing, the second part of the treatment has not yet been completed.
2. Fairy tales, for instance the tales of The Brothers Grimm, have frequent episodes characterized by oral aggression, at times even of cannibalism. (See "Little Red Riding Hood" where the wolf devours Grandmother, or "Hansel and Gretel," where the witch puts Hansel in the oven to be roasted.)

    Psychoanalytical theory has it that a child who becomes psychotic at an early age is likely to have been afflicted during the first oral psycho-sexual stage of development. The only area where I could hope to establish therapeutic contact with him was therefore in an area of oral conflict. Thus Grimm's fairy tales seemed a good choice.

    Another advantage of reading fairy tales was the fact that the oral conflicts here are too removed to cause anxiety but not to an extent where he would be unable to become emotionally engaged.
3. The scraping of the wax crayon with his finger nail was of an annihilating, aggressive nature, like grinding sand on the floor with one's shoe or crunching sand against the bottom of the sandbox with one's spade. Annihilating aggression of this kind would render him psychotically remote.
4. The narrative of this therapy is extremely condensed. A presentation of all the details would obscure the main issues.
5. He needed clearly defined guidelines for the use of fingerpaint so as not to become chaotic: painting within the limits of the paper, not using any more paint than what is needed for the presentation, not painting on himself or me, etc.
6. I use the term "devour" because I assume that for him the sense of impending doom or annihilation is closely connected to an archaic sensation of being devoured. In addition the term is easily demonstrated for him in body language.

    On other occasions when I could not be sure he

understood what I said, I would use body language, miming, dramatizing, demonstrations using the actual object, drawing, painting, etc.

A vivid description and a metapsychological image of what Punishing Iron experiences in this state of "devour or be devoured," is given by Haugsgjerd (Grunnlaget for en ny psykiatri, 1986) quoting Bion in his article on schizophrenia (1956):

"Splitting and projective identification assumes an excessive intensity, resulting in the population of the patient's mental world by strange, frightening and incomprehensible objects, "bizarre objects." Such bizarre objects are chaotic mixtures of projected ego-fragments, sensations, and objects which were already established*), which either "devour" or are "devoured" by the fragments ..."

* As far as "Iron" is concerned, these consist of part-objects and archaic pre-conceptions.

7. I sense that he is entering a symbiotic relationship with me, therefore all communication with him now is to be understood, not as questions or appeals, but rather as "mythical inductions."
8. An iron to him is a symbol associated with anxiety and compulsion, and it is a symbol which he has previously projected both at home and in school.
9. "The Evil Companion" is a projection of his merciless super-ego; which later, when the projection is abandoned, becomes the annihilating iron, "The Punishing Iron," in his belly, and eventually is externalized, "thrown up" into me for safer disposal.
10. It seems reasonable to view the emptying of the mug and the picture which follows immediately afterwards as two expressions of the same theme; an unconscious wish to assault his mother's body and appropriate the content of her body, including his father's penis.

Melanie Klein, in her studies of the earliest development of the oedipal complex, found that this unconscious wish goes into operation already at the time of weaning and is enhanced during potty-training, and that the uterus is

perceived to be the scene of all sexual processes and all development. ("Early stages of the oedipus conflict," 1928).
11. I assume that he, by throwing up the iron, (the merciless, punishing super-ego) as a part of the externalizing process, places it with, or transfers it to me. Through externalizing, the power of the cruel super-ego is reduced and his ego is strengthened relative to the sadistic id-impulse.
12. I had received information from school that he had been observed masturbating in front of a nude sculpture. Later he had expressed fears of losing his penis. His motions now in my office were of such a nature that I could be reasonably sure my suggestion was appropriate.
13. I show here his attempt to copy on paper a stick-construction to illustrate his great capacity for mechanical copying. In the light of this, his earlier "drawings of humans" (including his "self-portraits") also become understandable. I had for a long time suspected that these could only be mechanic projections of visual impressions, not renderings of something experienced, in that this would have been an impossibility.
14. Parallel to the therapeutic relationship to me he has a transference relationship to his two music therapists who, through jazz-inspired, improvisational music therapy lessons have helped enhance and expand the treatment considerably.

DISCUSSION

DIAGNOSTIC

Punishing Iron's development has been atypical since he was two years of age, perhaps even before that. Gradually his situation has developed into an autistic psychosis.

At the start of the treatment he is 13 years of age and his functioning is generally psychotic, also in a well structured school situation with a small, special group. He is living at home, attending school regularly where he is being tutored on a one-to-one basis and attending a small group when possible. His sister is two years younger and healthy.

He has developed some kind of a language, but uses it only in short messages, like "want drink", "need to go to bathroom", etc. More frequently he is using the language as a spontaneous break-through of psychotic anxiety-ridden exclamations: "Iron, twice as hot as the hottest thing in the world!", "am crazy!". Or he uses it for compulsive, repetitive inquiries: "What color is it?", "What do you get when you mix purple and yellow?"

At times, for instance when people's fear of him confirms and enhances his own fear, he clearly becomes hallucinated. In more structured situations he may be occupied with crayons or technical objects like cassettes, but in a compulsive manner. In such situations he displays an inner drive with the persevering strength of psychosis.

The short verbal messages and compulsive activity were small, positive signs, compared to the splitting and excessive projective identification — they opened up the way to the possibility of establishing a therapeutic line of communication.

Through music therapy he already found himself in a situation of communicating — using music. The music therapists had shown that he was able to create musical responses to their improvisations. It appears that he could use music to express feelings, and it was obvious that he had entered a positive transference situation with the therapists.

THERAPEUTIC GOAL

The least ambitious goal was that of establishing a therapeutic line of communication.

The next would have to be that of establishing a transference situation with him and finding a medium through which he could express himself symbolically.

The most comprehensive goal was, through cooperation with the music therapists, to carry out a long term therapy which would render him as non-psychotic as possible, and thus, more open for learning. It turned out later that it was possible to arrange for a long term project together with the school he attended, where he already received 2 – 3 music therapy lessons a week and 4 lessons a day of general tutoring.

THERAPEUTIC METHOD

This art interpretating therapy would have to be non-figurative, to a large extent based on colors and color combinations, and largely guided by a challenge to paint special themes. ("Prompted" pictures, see Introduction.)

In my view, this was a natural road to take — he did not draw figures (except for some copies); he was very interested in colors, and one could not expect a "free" picture production to begin with, due to a failing in general communication.

I could anticipate that his "messages", if therapeutic contact was established, would contain among other things experiences of "part-objects", thought elements from his earliest stages of development. Painting would offer him the possibility of expressing such experiences without using words, in the language of colors and shapes.

The musical and the pictorial modes of expression would mutually enhance each other.

Through interpretation of his graphic expression I would then strive to enable him to transfer his cruel, psychosis-provoking super-ego to me, establish a symbiotic contact situation and start up a gradual process of individuation. (Margaret Mahler, 1968.)

The therapeutic line of communication was established in 3 months through a reading of fairy tales by me, with graphic responses on his part.

The decisive element here was choice of themes. These would have to be of an oral-sadistic, cannibal nature. (See note 2 and 10 in narrative.) The presentation would have to be modulated according to his level of anxiety and the strength of the transference relationship. The dramatic rise before climax (roasting, devouring, biting, etc.) should ideally take place in a joint "crescendo", but I expected that the real situation in most cases would be me a little ahead, but open for retreat in the event that he became distant.

His graphic responses were at first very cautious, for instance with only a light increase of the pressure on the crayons; later heavier and more responsive to my encouragement. Such joint crescendos were often repeated: for instance from the moment right before the wolf is going to devour Grandmother to the actual time of devouring, over and over, with ever-increasing dramatic effect.

I believe it is important here to be aware of the fact that the aggression is in excess, the loading is in excess, and he will transfer a great deal before the therapist is found to be credible, that is, non-punishing.

A small, psychotic girl put it this way: "It felt good, hitting the floor, because it didn't hit me back!"

After this had taken place, the therapy developed along three lines: (1) the development of the transference situation; (2) the development of the content; and (3) the development of the artistic skill — the ability to keep within the limits, not letting a color invade the field of another, refrain from destroying the pictures by painting over them, etc.

(The testing out of the therapist's credibility was also carried out by means of a long line of tools like ball-point pens, scissors, hole puncher, stapler, that is, everything that can be used to annihilate in a sadistic manner.)

The first leap forward in the further development of the *transference* situation came with the introduction of my prohibition against his letting one color annihilate another. Then came the first direct attack on me, a forerunner of the negative transference situation.

The next leap came when I interpreted the connection between the iron (the terrible super-ego) and his confusion. This is symbolized by the fact that I become synonymous with his "Evil Companion." He attacks me by painting on my trousers.

The third leap came after I interpreted his infantile wish to annihilate the uterus and appropriate its content. This revelation enabled him to enter a symbiotic relationship with me.

The last leap came after an interpretation of the castration anxiety and his fear of punishment, whereupon he entered a period of new learning. And after a while he was able to put up the first, cautious line of separation between us as a symbol of an embryonic process of individuation.

The *themes* develop from initially revolving around the fact that one color devours another to later including that of specific colors having a distinct symbolic expressive content.

The phrase (or idea) "crazy" is altered and limited to "confused."

The shapes take on a magic meaning, the X'es stop time from running, a round field of a certain color becomes a breast symbol — another becomes a mouth, etc.

His *painting skills* develop from vertical lines to round shapes which attack each other. Here he takes a significant step when he manages to stay within specifically drawn borders. He is then allowed to mix colors rather than painting over colors.

The above establishes the groundwork for his next step: drawing his first, experienced human figures, himself and the therapists.

I believe the method so far has fulfilled the expectations that one had at the start of this therapy: The attempt to establish a line of communication and a therapeutic transference situation has been successful.

The further goal in terms of rendering him non-psychotic and available for further learning has been met in the therapy situation and largely so in the school situation. He is still somewhat unstable in the general education classes, but for long periods he is able to work constructively with the learning material without relapsing into compulsive activities.

The open anxiety and general psychotic behavior is gone, the tendency of the people around him to enhance his psychotic mechanisms is weakened, a fact which makes the social situation considerably easier.

LITERATURE

Alschuler, Rose H. & Hattwick, La Berta Weiss: Painting and Personality Vol. 2. The University of Chicago Press, Chicago, Illinois 1947.

Bredeli, Borghild: Tegning Fag Uttrykksmiddel Terapi, Tiden forlag, Oslo, 1982.

Bion, Wilfred R.: Seven Servants, J. Aronson, Inc., New York, N.Y. 1977.

Eriksen, Liv: Fra larve til sommerfugl: En separasjon-individuasjons-prosess belyst gjennom bilder fra en terapi. Hovedoppgave, Psykologisk Institutt, Oslo Universitet, 1986 (manus)

Freud, Anna: Normality and Pathology in Childhood. Assessment of Development. The Hogarth Press and Institute of Psychoanalysis, London 1966.
Freud, Sigmund: The collected Papers of Sigmund Freud, ed. Philip Rieff, Collier Books, New York, N.Y. 1963.
Freud, Sigmund: Drommetydning 1 and 2, J.W. Cappelen Forlag A/S, 1985.
Grotstein, James S. (ed): Do I Dare Disturb the Universe? Essays in Honor of W.R. Bion, Caesura Press, Los Angeles, 1982.
Haugsgjerd, Svein: Jaques Lacan og psykoanalysen, Gyldendal, Oslo 1986.
Haugsgjerd, Svein: Grunnlaget for en ny psykiatri. Pax forlag, Oslo 1986.
Klee, Paul: On Modern Art, Faber & Faber Ltd., London 1948.
Klein, Melanie et al.: Notes on some Schizoid Mechanisms, in Developments in Psychoanalysis, London, Hogarth Press, 1952.
Klein, Melanie: The Development of Mental Functioning, from Envy and Gratitude & Other Works, Delacorte Press/Seymour Lawrence, 1958.
Klein, Melanie: Contributions to Psycho-Analysis 1921 – 1945. Developments in child and adolescent psychology. McGraw-Hill Book Company. New York. Toronto. London, 1964.
Klein, Melanie: Heimann, P., and Money-Kyrle, R., New Directions in Psycho-Analysis. Tavistock Publications Ltd., 1955.
Klein Melanie: On the Origin of Transference, from Envy and Gratitude & Other Works 1946 – 1963. Delacorte Press/Seymour Lawrence, 1975.
Klein, Melanie: Narrative of a Child Analysis, Delacorte Press/Seymour Lawrence, 1975.
Kramer, Edith: Bildterapi med barn. Wahlstrom & Wickstrand, Stockholm, 1975.
Kramer, Edith: The Practice of Art Therapy with Children. American Journal of Art Therapy, 1972, 11, p. 89 – 110.
Kris, Ernst: Psychoanalytic explorations in Art. International University Press, Inc., New York, 1979.
Lewis, Noland D.C.: The practical value of Graphic Art in the Personality Studies. Psychoanalytical Revue, 1925, 12.

Lowenfeld, Viktor/Brittain, W.L.: Creative and Mental Growth, 3. ed., Macmillan Comp., New York, 1959.

Meltzer, Donald: The Kleinian Development, Clunie Press, Perthshire, 1978.

Munsterberg, Elisabeth: HFD-test. Psychological Evaluation of Children's Human Figure Drawings, Grune & Stratton, New York, London, 1968.

Mortensen, Karen Vibecke: Bornetegninger, udvikling og udtrykk. Munksgaard, Copenhagen, 1971.

Mahler, Margaret: On human Symbiosis and the Vicissitude of Individuation, International Universities Press, Inc., New York, 1968.

Naumburg, Margaret: An Introduction to Art Therapy, Teachers College Press, New York and London, 1973.

Naumburg, Margaret: Schizophrenic Art. Its meaning in Psychotherapy. Grune & Stratton, Inc., New York, 1950.

Naumburg, Margaret: Psychoneurotic Art, its Function in Psychotherapy, Grune & Stratton, Inc., New York, 1953.

Nævestad, Marie: The Colors of Rage and Love, Universitetsforlaget, Oslo, 1979.

Rubin, Judith Aron: Child Art Therapy. Van Nostrand Reinhold Comp., 1978.

Ruud, Even: Hva er musikkterapi? Gyldendal Forlag A/S, Oslo/Gjovik 1980.

Sandler, Joseph et al.: The Technique of Child Psychoanalysis. Discussions with Anna Freud. The Hogarth Press and the Institute of Psychoanalysis, London 1980.

Ude, Annelise, D.W.: Betty. Rapport fra en barnepsykiatrisk behandling. H. Ascheoug & Co., Oslo, 1978.

Winnicott, D.W.: Collected Papers. Tavistock Publications Ltd., London 1958.

BLUEBIRD

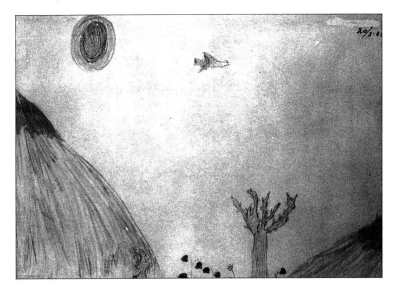

1

2

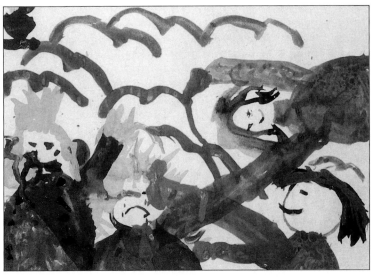

BLUEBIRD

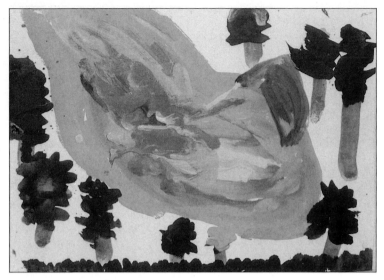

3

4

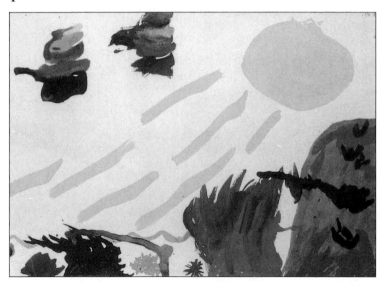

BLUEBIRD

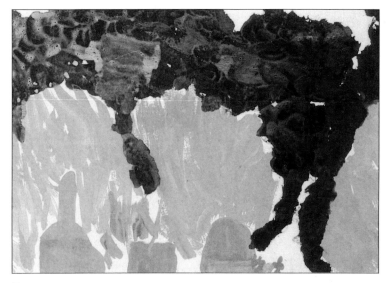

7

8

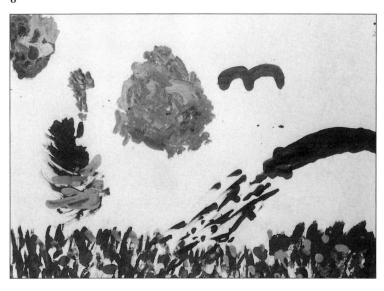

BLUEBIRD

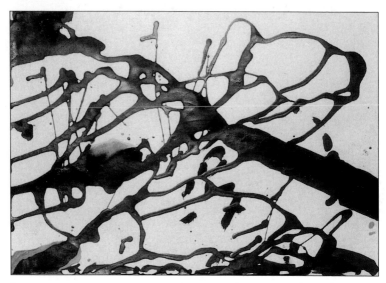

9

11

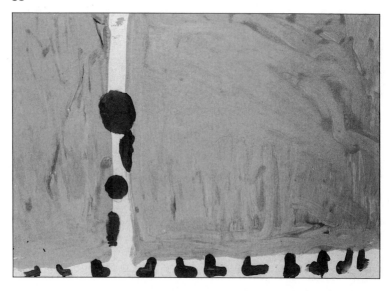

BLUEBIRD

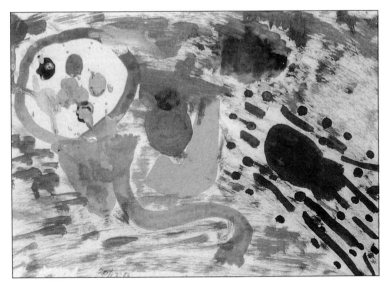

12

13

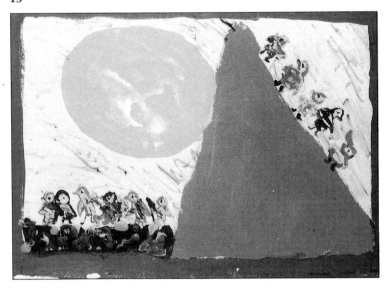

BLUEBIRD

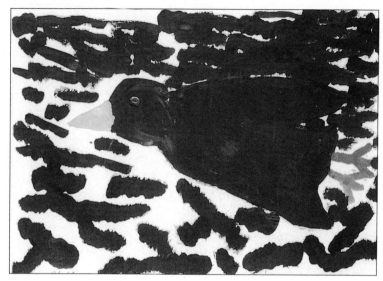

14

15

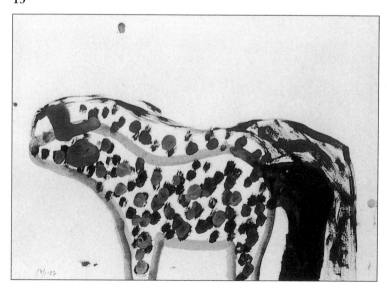

BLUEBIRD

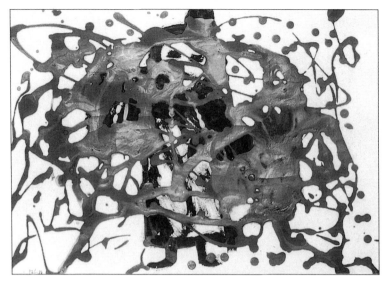

16

18

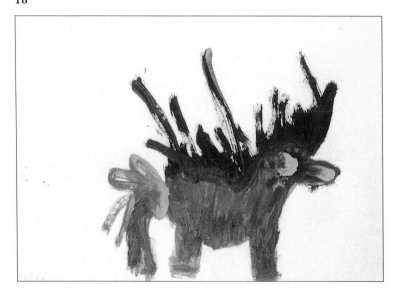

BLUEBIRD

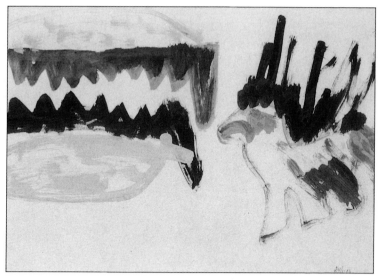

19

20

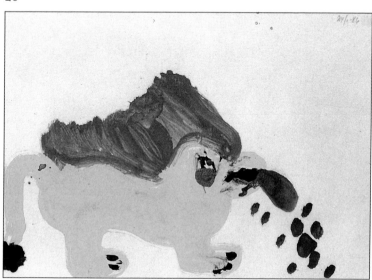

BLUEBIRD

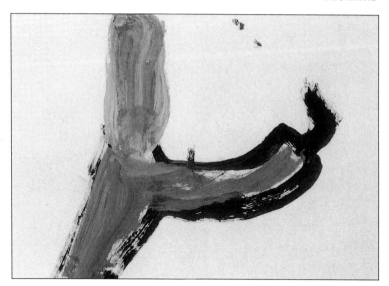

25

28

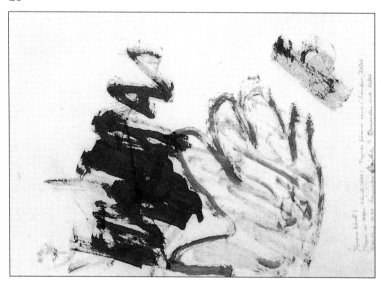

BLUEBIRD

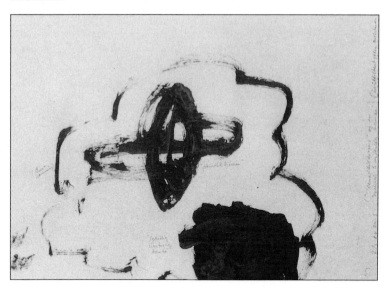

30

32

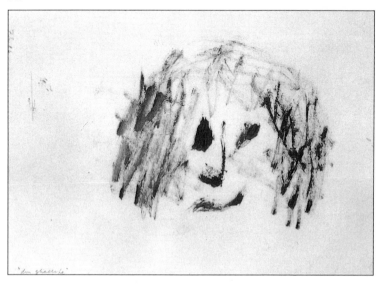

BLUEBIRD

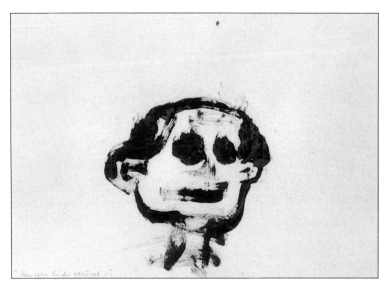

33

35

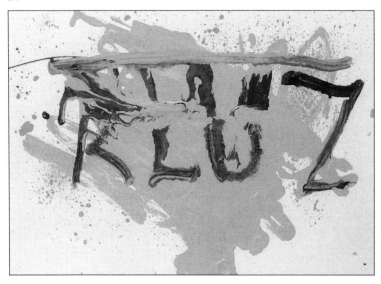

BLUEBIRD

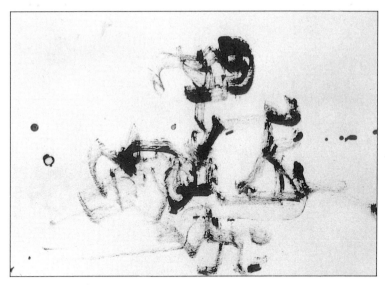

41

42

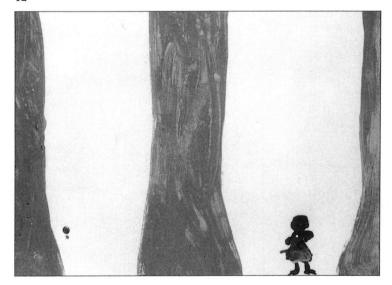

BLUEBIRD

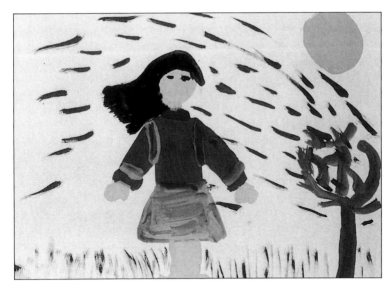

47

49

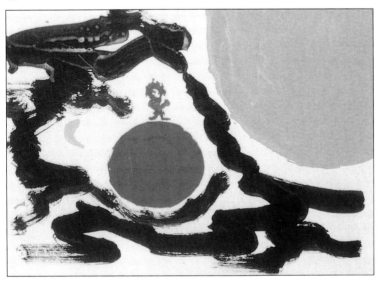

BLUEBIRD

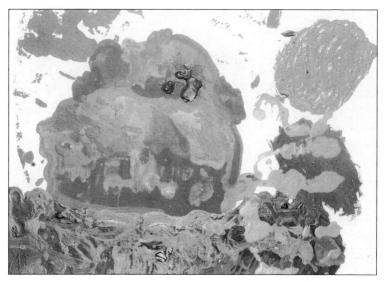

51

52

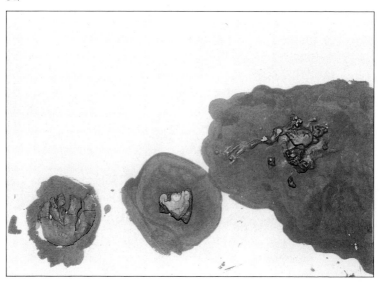

BLUEBIRD

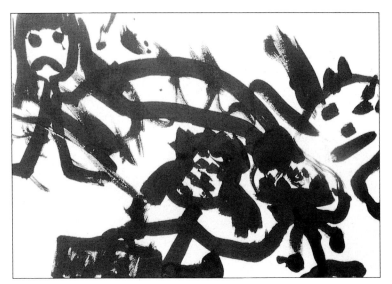

53

54

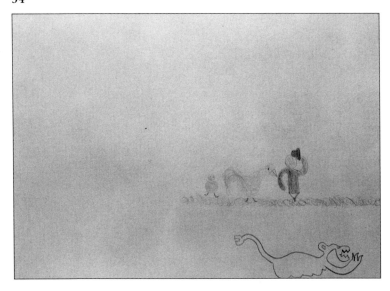

BLUEBIRD

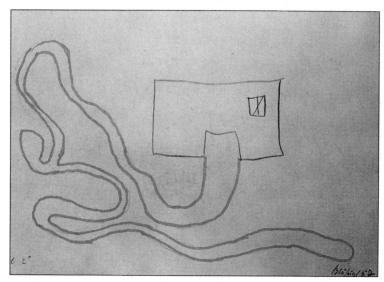

57

58

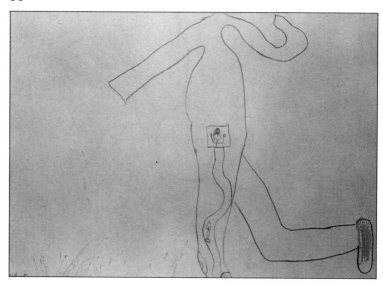

BLUEBIRD

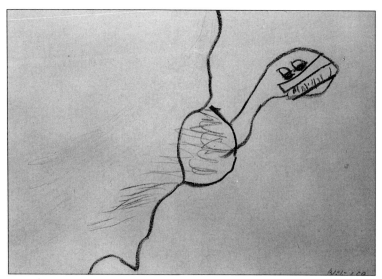

59

60

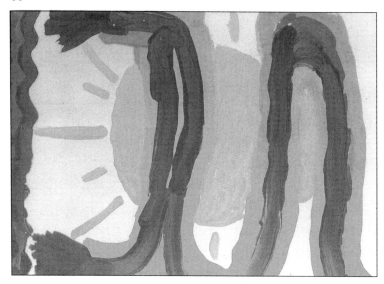

BLUEBIRD

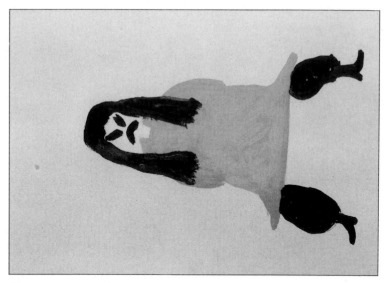

61

62

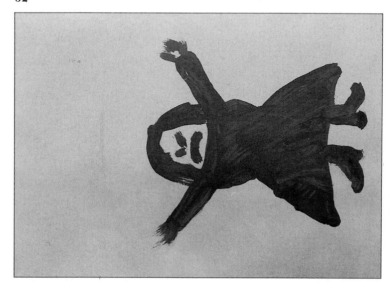

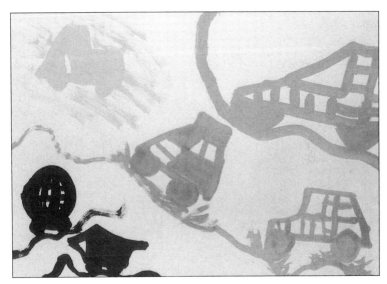

63

64

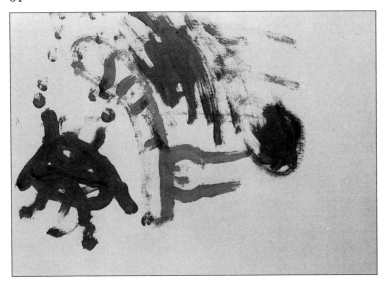

BLUEBIRD

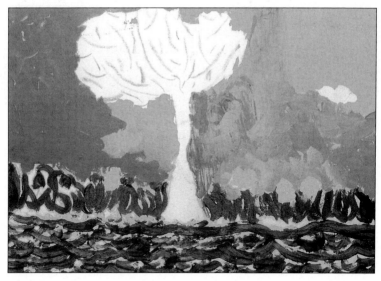

ROCKET

1

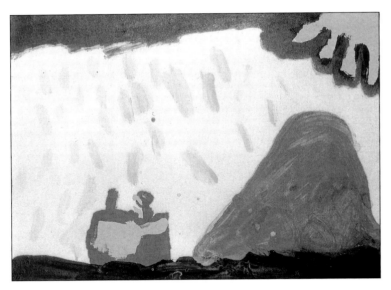

2

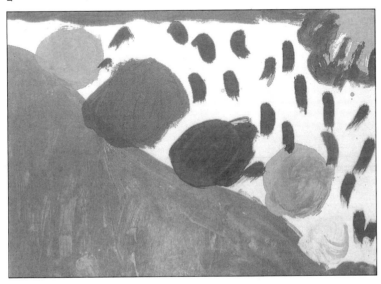

ROCKET

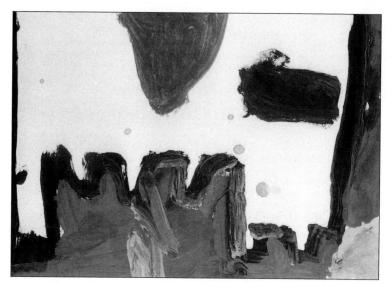

3

4

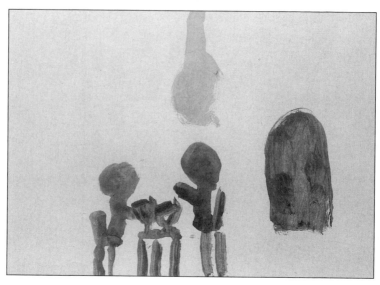

ROCKET

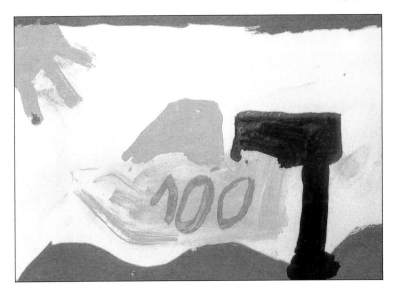

5

6

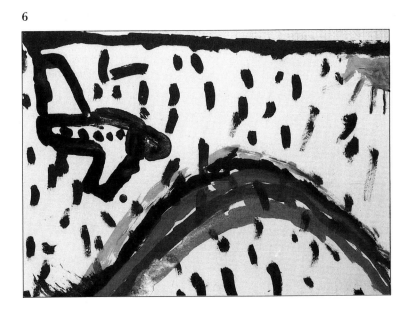

ROCKET

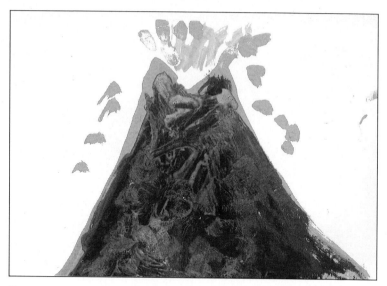

7

12

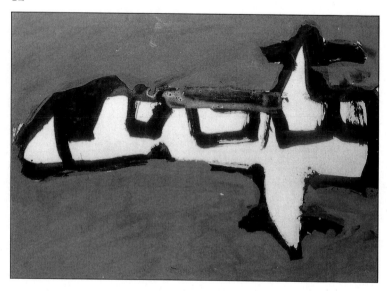

ROCKET

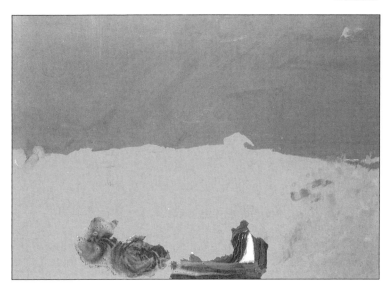

15

17

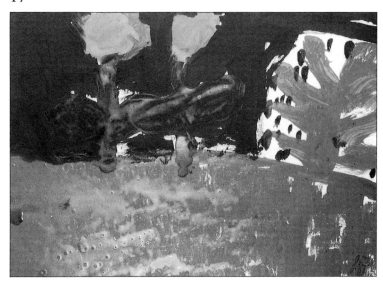

ROCKET

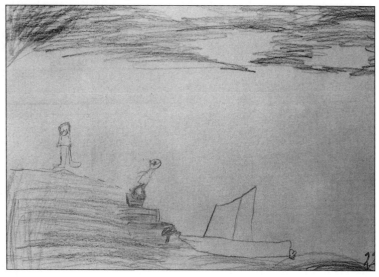

22

25

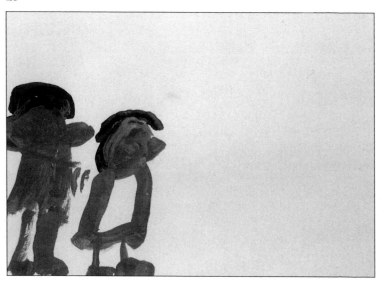

ROCKET

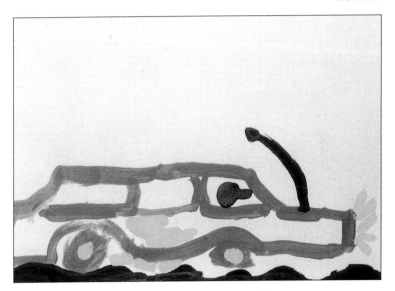

26

27

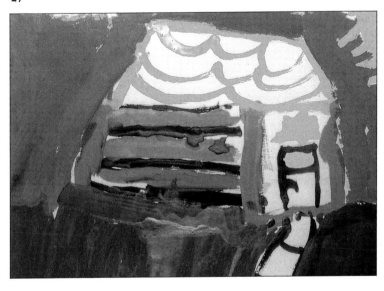

ROCKET

28

30

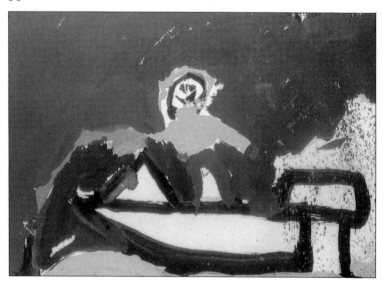

ROCKET

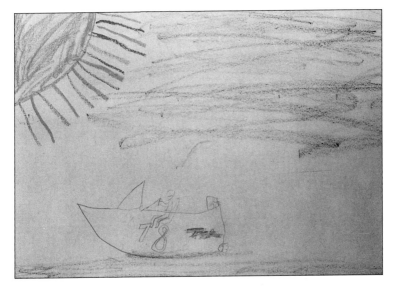

35

36

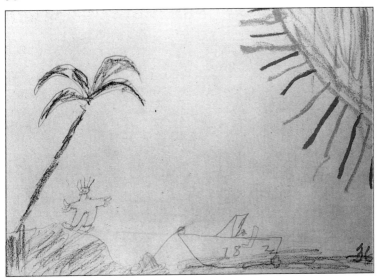

ROCKET

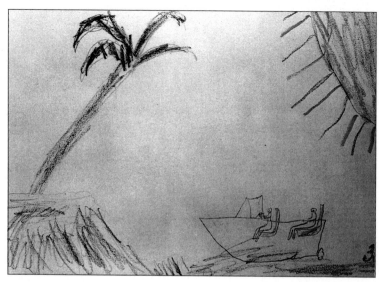

38

BLACK RHOMB

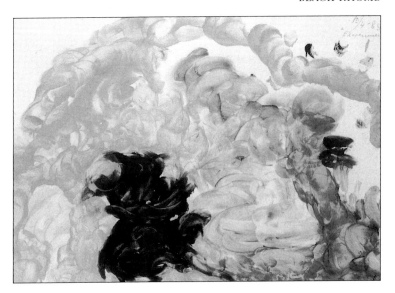

1

2

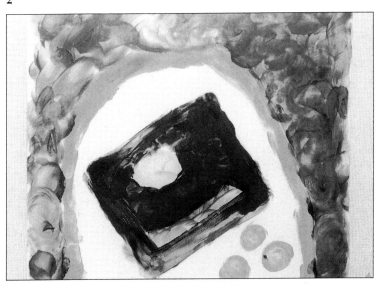

BLACK RHOMB

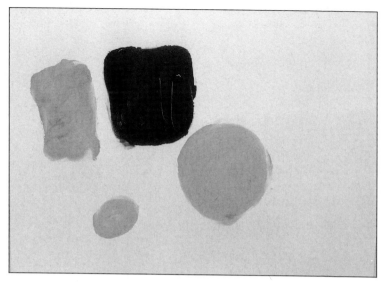

3

4

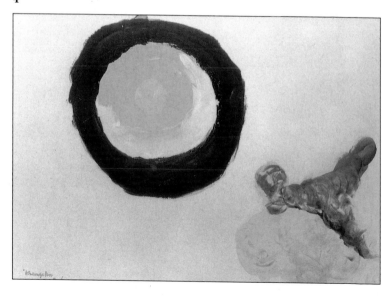

BLACK RHOMB

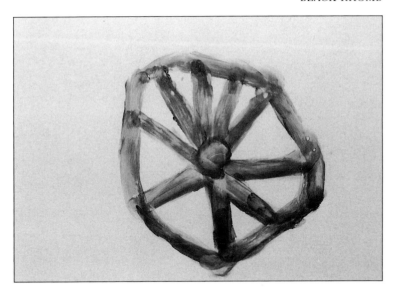

5

6

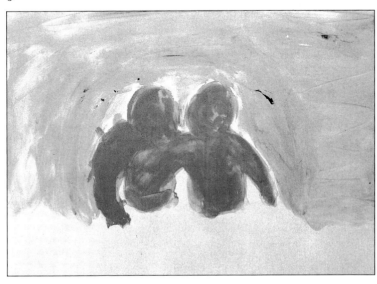

BLACK RHOMB

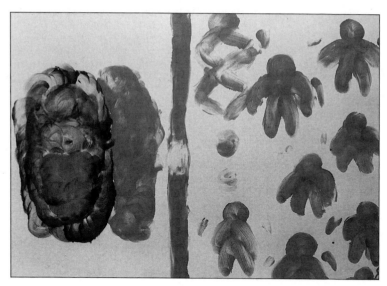

8

15

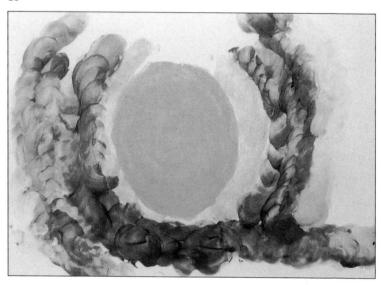

BLACK RHOMB

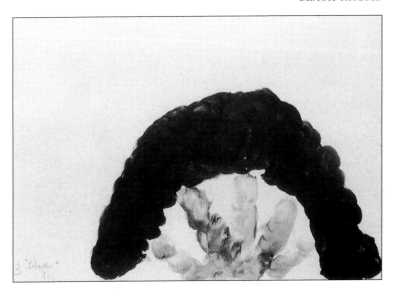

16

18

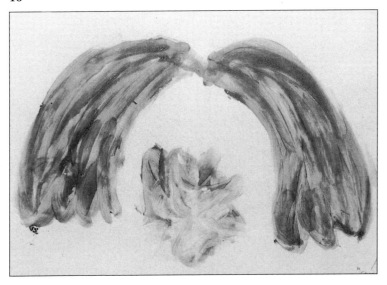

BLACK RHOMB

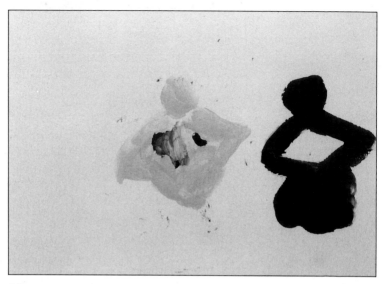

23

24

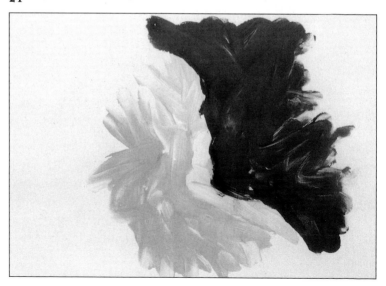

BLACK RHOMB

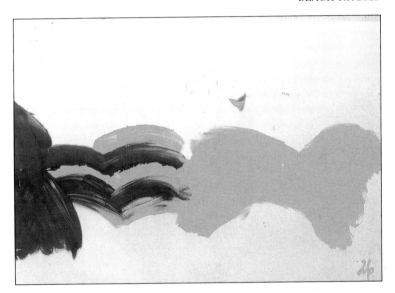

26

28

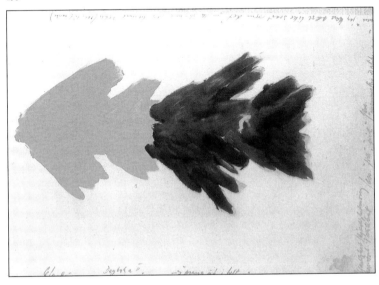

BLACK RHOMB

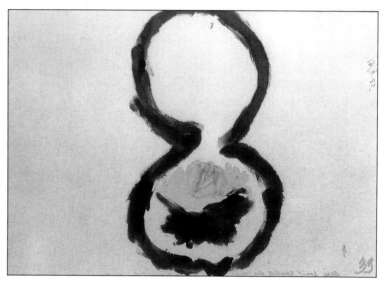

33

34

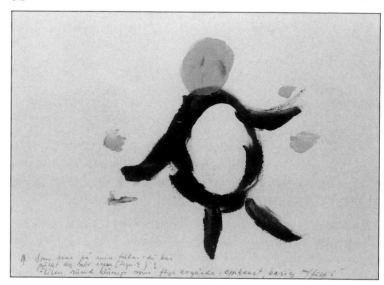

BLACK RHOMB

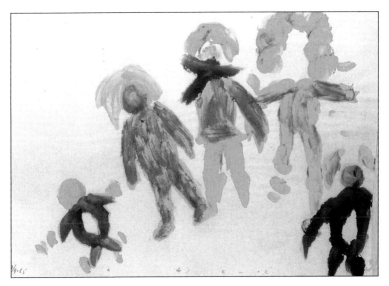

35

36

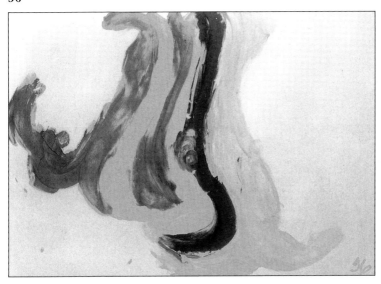

EAGLE

1

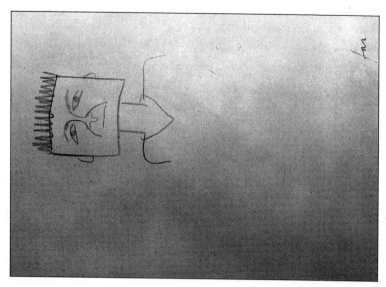

2

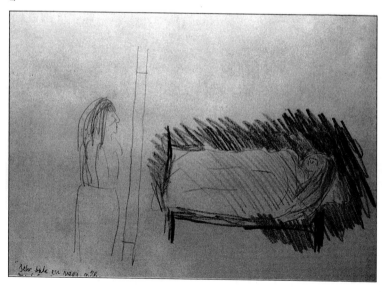

EAGLE

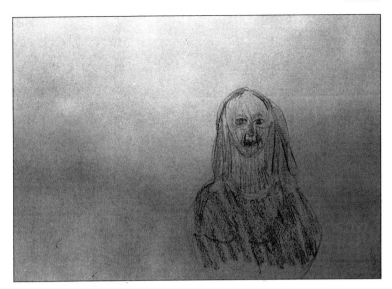

3

4

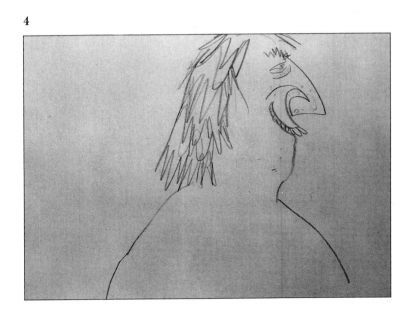

EAGLE

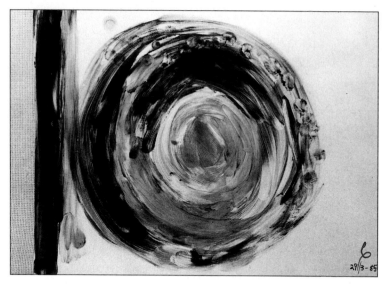

6

7

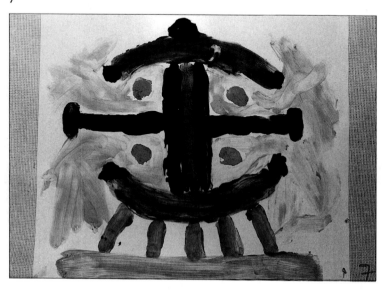

EAGLE

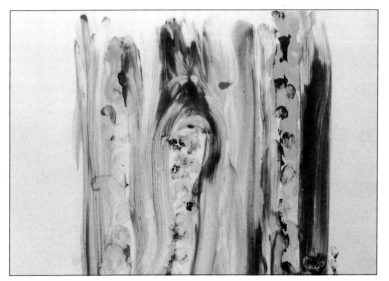

10

11

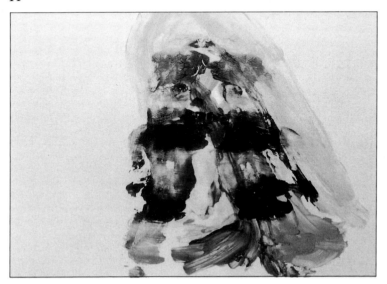

EAGLE

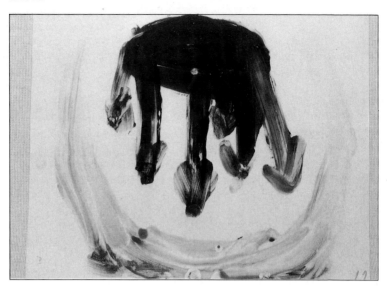

12

13

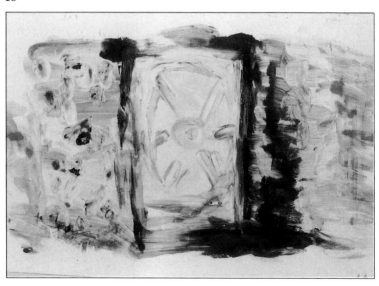

EAGLE

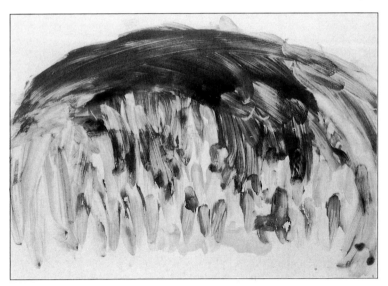

14

15

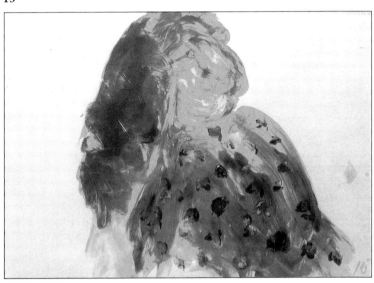

EAGLE

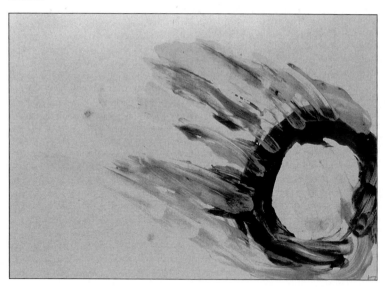

17

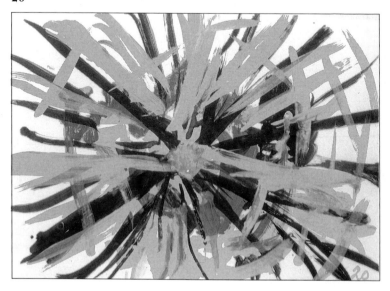

20

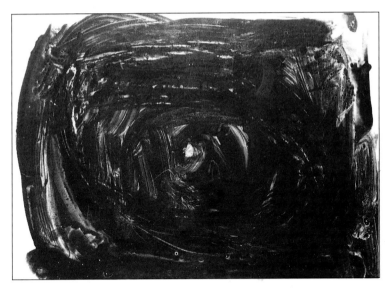

21

29

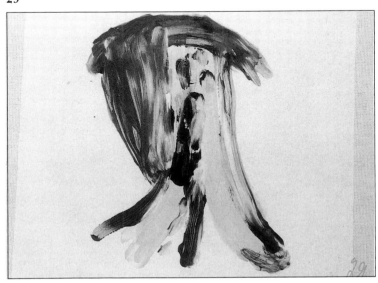

EAGLE

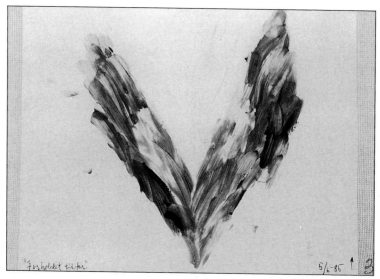

36

37

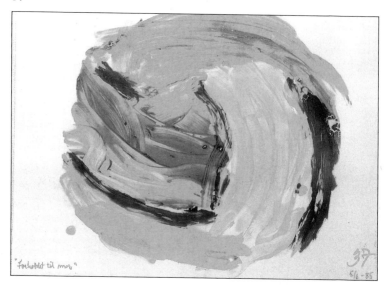

EAGLE

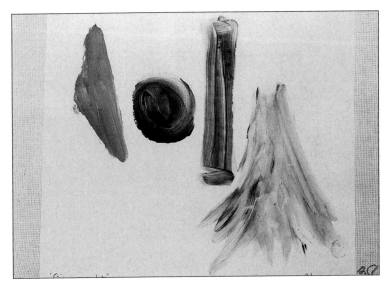

38

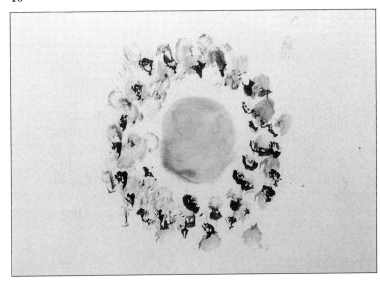

40

EAGLE

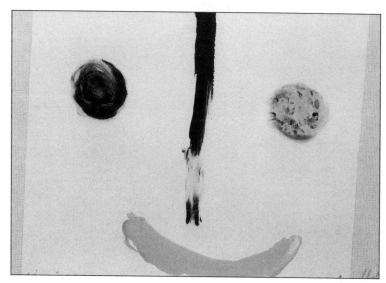

41

PUNISHING IRON

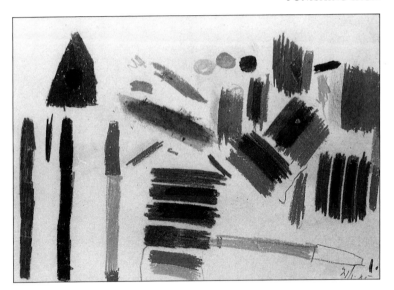

1

2

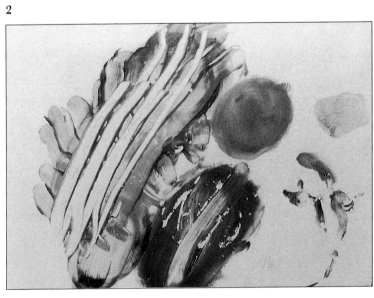

PUNISHING IRON

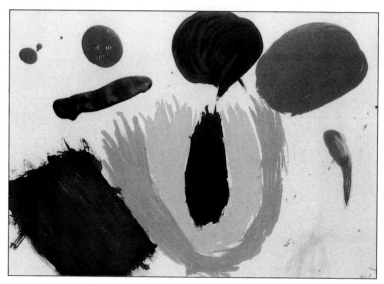

3

5

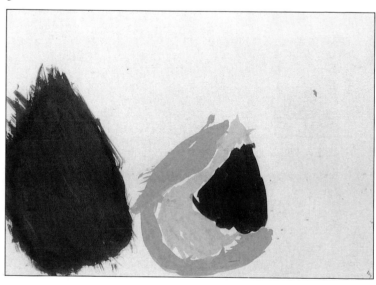

PUNISHING IRON

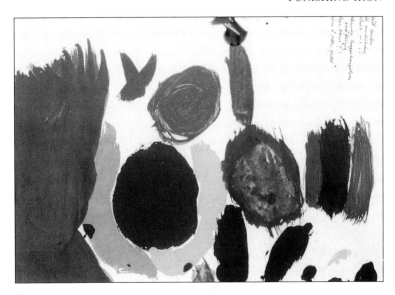

6

8

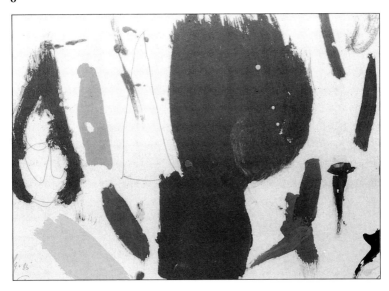

PUNISHING IRON

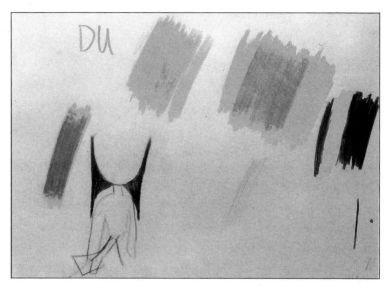

11

15

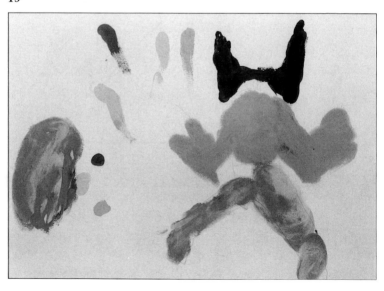

PUNISHING IRON

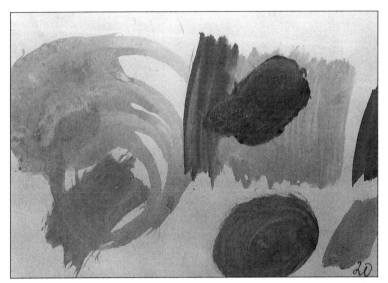

20

21

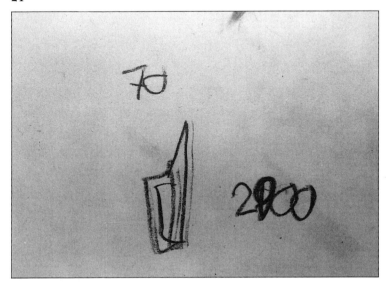

PUNISHING IRON

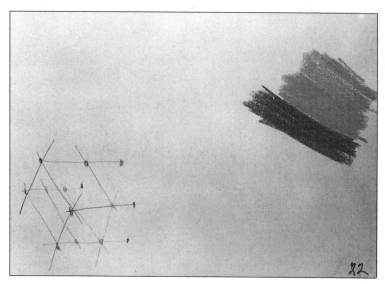

22

23

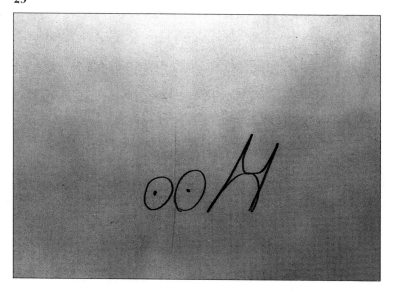

PUNISHING IRON

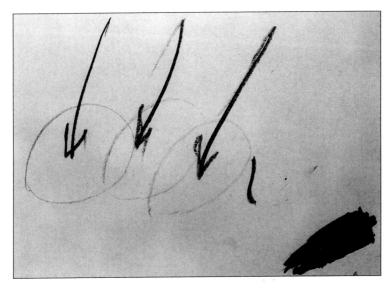

24

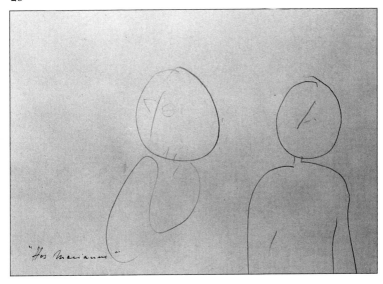

25

PUNISHING IRON

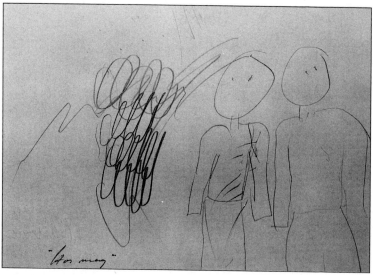